Living With Diabetes

as an Adult

Empowering Strategies for Managing, Thriving, and Living a Fulfilling Life Amidst the Challenges of Diabetes

CATHERINE CLARKSON

Table of Contents

Introduction: Navigating Life with Diabetes as an Adult

Living with diabetes is a journey that millions of adults around the world embark upon every day. It's a path filled with challenges, triumphs, and a constant need for balance. In this book, we will delve into the intricacies of navigating life with diabetes as an adult, providing insights, practical advice, and empowering strategies to help you not only manage the condition but thrive despite its challenges.

Understanding Diabetes

To navigate life with diabetes, it's crucial to first understand the nature of the condition. Diabetes is a chronic health disorder that occurs when the body cannot produce enough insulin or effectively use the insulin it produces. Insulin is a hormone that regulates blood sugar, and without it, the balance of glucose in the bloodstream is disrupted. This disruption leads to elevated blood sugar levels, which, if not managed, can result in various health complications.

Types of Diabetes

Beyond the general classification of Type 1 and Type 2 diabetes, this section delves into less common forms, such as gestational diabetes and prediabetes. Exploring these variations is crucial for a comprehensive understanding, as they require tailored approaches to management. We discuss risk factors, diagnostic criteria, and potential lifestyle modifications for each subtype.

Importance of Diabetes Management

The journey of living with diabetes begins with recognizing its significance. Effective management is not only about controlling blood sugar levels but also preventing complications that can impact various organs, such as the heart, kidneys, and eyes. This section underscores the importance of proactive management, emphasizing the role it plays in ensuring a fulfilling and healthy life despite the diagnosis.

Effective diabetes management is the key to leading a fulfilling life with the condition. Managing diabetes involves a multifaceted approach, encompassing lifestyle changes, medication, and regular monitoring. The importance of proactive management cannot be overstated, as it directly impacts one's overall well-being.

This book aims to be your guide through the intricacies of diabetes management. Whether you are newly diagnosed or have been living with diabetes for years, there is always room for learning and improvement. We will explore various aspects of managing diabetes, from understanding insulin and blood glucose monitoring to the significance of a well-balanced diet and regular physical activity.

Embarking on the Diabetes Journey

Getting diagnosed with diabetes can be a life-altering experience. It often comes with a range of emotions, including shock, denial, and fear of the unknown. In the chapter on diagnosis and treatment, we will explore what it means to receive a diabetes diagnosis and the initial steps you can take to navigate this new chapter in your life. From understanding treatment options to exploring medications and insulin, we will address the various components of diabetes care.

Nutrition and Diet

One of the cornerstones of effective diabetes management is adopting a healthy and balanced diet. Food choices play a crucial role in regulating blood sugar levels, and understanding how different foods impact your body is essential. In the section on nutrition and diet, we will delve into the principles of a diabetes-friendly diet, covering topics such as carbohydrate counting, meal planning, and practical tips for making healthier food choices.

Physical Activity

Regular physical activity is not only beneficial for overall health but is also a key component of diabetes management. Engaging in exercise helps improve insulin sensitivity and promotes weight management. In the chapter on physical activity, we will explore the relationship between exercise and diabetes, guiding creating a fitness routine that suits your lifestyle and addressing common barriers to staying active.

Blood Sugar Management

Understanding and managing blood sugar levels are fundamental aspects of living with diabetes. In this section, we will discuss the significance of monitoring blood sugar levels, recognizing the symptoms of hypoglycemia (low blood sugar) and hyperglycemia (high blood sugar), and strategies for maintaining optimal blood sugar control.

Managing Stress and Mental Health

The relationship between stress and diabetes is intricate. Stress can affect blood sugar levels and make diabetes management more challenging. In the chapter on managing stress and mental health, we will explore the connection between stress and diabetes, providing practical coping strategies and highlighting the importance of seeking support from healthcare professionals and loved ones.

Monitoring and Regular Check-ups

Regular check-ups and monitoring are essential components of diabetes care. Timely visits to healthcare providers, coupled with regular monitoring of blood sugar levels and other health parameters, contribute to effective diabetes management. We will discuss the importance of regular check-ups, offer guidance on self-monitoring, and emphasize the value of clear communication with healthcare providers.

Living a Full and Active Life

While living with diabetes poses its share of challenges, it should not hinder your ability to lead a full and active life. In this section, we will explore strategies for overcoming challenges, address topics such as traveling with diabetes, and discuss the impact of the condition on relationships. Living a fulfilling life with diabetes is not only possible but achievable with the right mindset and tools.

Future Developments and Research

The field of diabetes research is continually evolving, with ongoing efforts to develop new treatments and improve existing ones. In this chapter, we will explore emerging treatments, current research initiatives, and the hope for future advancements in diabetes care. Staying informed about the latest developments can empower individuals living with diabetes to make informed decisions about their healthcare.

Resources for Living with Diabetes

Access to reliable information and support is crucial for effectively managing diabetes. In this chapter, we will provide a comprehensive list of resources, including diabetes associations, recommended books and websites, and information about support groups and communities. Having a strong support network and access to accurate information can significantly enhance your ability to navigate life with diabetes.

Conclusion

In the concluding chapter, we will summarize the key insights and takeaways from the book. Embracing a healthy lifestyle and taking control of your diabetes journey are empowering steps toward living a fulfilling life as an adult with diabetes. Remember, while diabetes is a part of your life, it does not define who you are. With knowledge, support, and determination, you can navigate the challenges and embrace the opportunities that lie ahead.

Chapter 1: Understanding Diabetes: Types, Causes, and Complications

Overview of Diabetes Types: Type 1, Type 2, and Gestational Diabetes

Diabetes is a complex and chronic health condition characterized by elevated blood sugar levels. Understanding the different types of diabetes is crucial for effective management and tailored care. In this section, we will delve into the distinctive features of Type 1 diabetes, Type 2 diabetes, and gestational diabetes.

Type 1 Diabetes: Unraveling the Autoimmune Connection

Type 1 diabetes is an autoimmune condition where the immune system mistakenly attacks and destroys the insulin-producing cells in the pancreas. This results in a deficiency of insulin, a hormone vital for regulating blood sugar levels. Typically diagnosed in childhood or adolescence, Type 1 diabetes accounts for about 5-10% of all diabetes cases.

The exact cause of Type 1 diabetes remains elusive, but genetic predisposition and environmental factors are believed to play a role. Individuals with Type 1 diabetes require insulin injections or an insulin pump to manage their blood sugar levels effectively. Understanding the unique challenges of living with Type 1 diabetes is essential for individuals, their families, and healthcare providers.

Type 2 Diabetes: Lifestyle and Genetic Factors

Type 2 diabetes is the more prevalent form of diabetes, accounting for approximately 90-95% of cases. Unlike Type 1 diabetes, Type 2 diabetes is often linked to lifestyle factors such as poor diet, lack of physical activity, and obesity. Genetic factors also contribute to the risk of developing Type 2 diabetes.

In Type 2 diabetes, the body either doesn't produce enough insulin or becomes resistant to its effects, leading to elevated blood sugar levels. While it often occurs in adulthood, an increasing number of cases are being diagnosed in children and adolescents due to rising obesity rates. Management of Type 2 diabetes involves lifestyle modifications, oral medications, and, in some cases, insulin therapy.

Gestational Diabetes: Navigating Pregnancy and Beyond

Gestational diabetes develops during pregnancy and affects about 2-10% of pregnant women. It occurs when the body cannot produce enough insulin to meet the increased demands of pregnancy. While gestational diabetes usually resolves after childbirth, it poses risks to both the mother and the baby.

Untreated gestational diabetes can lead to complications during pregnancy and delivery, as well as an increased risk of Type 2 diabetes for both the mother and the child later in life. Managing gestational diabetes involves monitoring blood sugar levels, adopting a healthy diet, and in some cases, using insulin. Comprehensive prenatal care and postpartum follow-up are crucial for the well-being of both mother and child.

Understanding the nuances of each diabetes type allows individuals and healthcare professionals to tailor treatment plans, support strategies, and education efforts to meet specific needs.

Understanding the Causes and Risk Factors of Diabetes

Delving into the causes and risk factors of diabetes provides valuable insights into the prevention and management of this prevalent health condition. From genetic predisposition to lifestyle choices, various factors contribute to the development of diabetes.

Genetic Predisposition: Unraveling the Family Connection

Genetics plays a significant role in diabetes risk. Individuals with a family history of diabetes, especially those with close relatives like parents or siblings with the condition, are at a higher risk of developing diabetes themselves. Specific genes associated with insulin production and glucose metabolism contribute to this familial link.

While having a family history of diabetes increases the risk, it doesn't guarantee that an individual will develop the condition. Genetic factors interact with environmental influences, highlighting the importance of a holistic approach to understanding diabetes risk.

Lifestyle Factors: Diet, Physical Activity, and Obesity

The modern lifestyle, characterized by sedentary behavior and unhealthy dietary choices, has led to a significant increase in Type 2 diabetes cases. Poor nutrition, particularly diets high in processed foods, saturated fats, and added sugars, contributes to obesity and insulin resistance.

Regular physical activity plays a crucial role in diabetes prevention and management. Exercise improves insulin sensitivity, helps control weight, and promotes overall well-being. Sedentary lifestyles, on the other hand, contribute to weight gain and increase the risk of developing Type 2 diabetes.

Obesity: The Link Between Body Weight and Diabetes

Obesity is a well-established risk factor for Type 2 diabetes. Excess body fat, especially abdominal fat, contributes to insulin resistance, where the body's cells do not respond effectively to insulin. This resistance leads to elevated blood sugar levels.

Addressing obesity through lifestyle modifications, including a balanced diet and regular exercise, is a key component of diabetes prevention. Weight loss interventions have been shown to improve insulin sensitivity and reduce the risk of developing Type 2 diabetes.

Age and Ethnicity: Exploring Demographic Factors

Age and ethnicity also play a role in diabetes risk. While Type 1 diabetes is often diagnosed in children and young adults, Type 2 diabetes is more common in older individuals. The risk of developing Type 2 diabetes increases with age, especially after the age of 45.

Certain ethnic groups, including African Americans, Hispanic Americans, Native Americans, and Asian Americans, have a higher predisposition to diabetes. Genetic factors and disparities in healthcare access and socioeconomic status contribute to these variations in diabetes prevalence among different ethnicities.

Gestational Diabetes: Pregnancy-Related Risk Factor

Gestational diabetes, occurring during pregnancy, is a unique risk factor for both the mother and the child. Women who have had gestational diabetes are at an increased risk of developing Type 2 diabetes later in life. Additionally, children born to mothers with gestational diabetes have a higher risk of obesity and Type 2 diabetes.

Understanding these causes and risk factors provides a foundation for targeted prevention efforts and personalized healthcare strategies. Lifestyle modifications, regular screenings, and early intervention can significantly reduce the risk of developing diabetes and its associated complications.

Potential Complications and Long-term Effects of Diabetes

Living with diabetes requires constant vigilance and proactive management to prevent and mitigate potential complications. Diabetes can affect various organs and systems in the body, leading to both short-term and long-term complications.

Cardiovascular Complications: Navigating Heart Health

Individuals with diabetes have an increased risk of cardiovascular complications, including heart disease and stroke. Elevated blood sugar levels contribute to the buildup of fatty deposits in the blood vessels, leading to atherosclerosis. Additionally, diabetes can affect cholesterol levels and blood pressure, further increasing the risk of heart-related issues.

Managing diabetes involves not only controlling blood sugar levels but also addressing other cardiovascular risk factors. Lifestyle modifications, such as adopting a heart-healthy diet and engaging in regular physical activity, are essential for preventing cardiovascular complications.

Neuropathy: Understanding Nerve Damage

Diabetic neuropathy is a common complication characterized by nerve damage. It often affects the peripheral nerves, leading to symptoms such as tingling, numbness, and pain, usually starting in the feet and gradually progressing to other areas of the body.

Proactive management of diabetes, including blood sugar control and regular foot care, is crucial for preventing and managing neuropathy. Early detection and intervention can help slow the progression of nerve damage and improve overall quality of life.

Nephropathy: Kidney Health and Diabetes

Diabetes is a leading cause of kidney disease, known as diabetic nephropathy. Elevated blood sugar levels can damage the small blood vessels in the kidneys, leading to impaired kidney function. If left untreated, diabetic nephropathy can progress to end-stage renal disease, necessitating dialysis or kidney transplantation.

Regular monitoring of kidney function through blood and urine tests is essential for individuals with diabetes. Blood pressure control, maintaining healthy blood sugar levels, and adopting a kidney-friendly diet contribute to kidney health.

Retinopathy: Preserving Vision

Diabetic retinopathy is a diabetes complication affecting the eyes. It involves damage to the blood vessels in the retina, leading to vision impairment and, in severe cases, blindness. Regular eye examinations and early intervention are critical for preventing and managing diabetic retinopathy.

Blood sugar control, blood pressure management, and routine eye screenings are integral components of preserving vision in individuals with diabetes. Timely treatment, including laser therapy or surgery, may be recommended in advanced cases.

Foot Complications: Importance of Foot Care

Foot complications are common in individuals with diabetes due to reduced blood flow and nerve damage. Peripheral neuropathy can lead to reduced sensation in the feet, making individuals less aware of injuries or infections. Poor circulation further complicates the healing process.

Daily foot care, including regular inspection, moisturizing, and proper footwear, is essential for preventing foot complications. Prompt attention to any signs of infection or injury can prevent serious issues and potential amputations.

Mental Health: Addressing the Emotional Impact

The emotional impact of living with diabetes should not be underestimated. The constant need for monitoring, lifestyle adjustments, and the potential for complications can contribute to stress, anxiety, and depression. Mental health support is a crucial aspect of comprehensive diabetes care.

Open communication with healthcare providers, seeking support from friends and family, and considering counseling or support groups can help individuals cope with the emotional challenges of diabetes. A holistic approach to diabetes care includes addressing both the physical and emotional aspects of well-being.

Understanding these potential complications emphasizes the importance of proactive diabetes management. Regular medical check-ups, adherence to prescribed treatments, and lifestyle modifications are key strategies for preventing and mitigating the long-term effects of diabetes.

Chapter 2: Managing Blood Sugar Levels: Monitoring and Medications

Blood Glucose Monitoring: Techniques and Tools

Effective blood glucose monitoring is a cornerstone of successful diabetes management. Regular monitoring provides valuable insights into how lifestyle choices, medications, and other factors impact blood sugar levels. In this section, we will explore various techniques and tools available for blood glucose monitoring.

Self-Monitoring of Blood Glucose (SMBG): Empowering Individuals

Self-monitoring of blood glucose (SMBG) is a vital component of diabetes management, putting individuals in control of their daily health. SMBG involves using a blood glucose meter to measure blood sugar levels at home. The process typically includes pricking a fingertip to obtain a small blood sample, which is then applied to a test strip and inserted into the meter for analysis.

Regular SMBG allows individuals to track their blood sugar levels throughout the day, identifying patterns and making informed decisions about medication, diet, and physical activity. It is especially crucial for those using insulin or other medications that may cause fluctuations in blood sugar levels.

Advancements in technology have led to the development of continuous glucose monitoring (CGM) systems, which provide real-time data on blood sugar levels. CGM involves placing a small sensor under the skin, usually on the abdomen, to continuously measure glucose levels throughout the day and night. The sensor transmits data wirelessly to a device or smartphone, offering a comprehensive view of blood sugar trends.

Choosing the Right Blood Glucose Meter: Factors to Consider

Selecting the right blood glucose meter is essential for accurate and convenient monitoring. Various meters are available on the market, each with its features and capabilities. When choosing a meter, consider the following factors:

1. **Accuracy:** Look for a meter with proven accuracy. Check reviews, and consult with healthcare providers to ensure the selected meter provides reliable results.

2. **Ease of Use:** A user-friendly meter with clear instructions and a simple testing process can make monitoring less daunting. Consider features like large buttons, backlight, and audible alerts.

3. **Size and Portability:** Choose a meter that fits your lifestyle. Compact and portable meters are convenient for on-the-go monitoring.

4. **Data Storage:** Some meters come with built-in memory or connect to apps to store and analyze historical data. This feature can be beneficial for tracking trends over time.

5. **Cost and Insurance Coverage:** Consider the cost of the meter and the availability of insurance coverage for supplies such as test strips. Some insurance plans may cover specific brands or models.

6. **Connectivity:** Meters with Bluetooth or other connectivity options allow seamless data transfer to smartphones or other devices, facilitating easier data management and sharing with healthcare providers.

Frequency of Blood Glucose Monitoring: Tailoring to Individual Needs

The frequency of blood glucose monitoring varies among individuals and is often determined by factors such as the type of diabetes, treatment plan, and overall health. Healthcare providers typically recommend specific testing times, which may include:

1. **Fasting Blood Sugar:** Measured in the morning before eating or drinking anything, fasting blood sugar levels provide baseline information on how the body manages glucose overnight.

2. **Postprandial Blood Sugar:** Measured 1-2 hours after meals, postprandial testing helps assess how the body responds to specific foods and aids in meal planning.

3. **Before and After Exercise:** Monitoring blood sugar levels before and after physical activity is essential, as exercise can impact glucose levels. It helps individuals understand the need for adjustments in medication or food intake.

4. **Before Bed:** Nighttime monitoring is crucial for individuals at risk of nocturnal hypoglycemia or those experiencing unexplained fluctuations in blood sugar levels during sleep.

5. **Periodic Checks:** In addition to routine testing, periodic checks throughout the day can help identify trends and patterns, enabling more personalized and effective diabetes management.

Establishing a routine for blood glucose monitoring, based on individual needs and healthcare provider recommendations, empowers individuals to actively manage their diabetes and make informed decisions about their daily activities.

Medications for Diabetes Management

Medications play a pivotal role in diabetes management, helping control blood sugar levels and reduce the risk of complications. The choice of medications depends on the type of diabetes, individual health factors, and treatment goals. In this section, we will explore the various classes of medications used in diabetes management.

Oral Medications: Improving Insulin Sensitivity and Production

Oral medications are commonly prescribed for individuals with Type 2 diabetes. They work through different mechanisms to lower blood sugar levels. Some of the main classes of oral medications include:

1. **Metformin:** Metformin is often the first-line medication for Type 2 diabetes. It improves insulin sensitivity, reduces glucose production in the liver, and enhances glucose uptake by cells.

2. **Sulfonylureas:** These medications stimulate the pancreas to release more insulin. They include drugs like glipizide, glyburide, and glimepiride.

3. **Dipeptidyl Peptidase-4 (DPP-4) Inhibitors:** DPP-4 inhibitors enhance the body's natural ability to lower blood sugar levels by increasing the concentration of incretin hormones. Examples include sitagliptin and saxagliptin.

4. **Thiazolidinediones (TZDs):** TZDs improve insulin sensitivity in muscle and fat cells. Rosiglitazone and pioglitazone are examples of TZDs.

5. **SGLT-2 Inhibitors:** Sodium-glucose co-transporter 2 (SGLT-2) inhibitors reduce blood sugar levels by increasing the excretion of glucose in the urine. Canagliflozin, dapagliflozin, and empagliflozin belong to this class.

6. **GLP-1 Receptor Agonists:** Glucagon-like peptide-1 (GLP-1) receptor agonists stimulate insulin secretion and reduce glucagon production. They also slow down gastric emptying, leading to improved blood sugar control. Examples include exenatide and liraglutide.

Injectable Medications: Enhancing Insulin Management

For individuals with Type 1 diabetes and some with Type 2 diabetes, injectable medications are often necessary to supplement or replace natural insulin production. These medications include:

1. **Rapid-Acting Insulin:** These insulins work quickly to lower blood sugar levels and are typically taken just before or after meals. Examples include insulin lispro, insulin aspart, and insulin glulisine.

2. **Short-Acting Insulin:** Short-acting insulins take effect within 30 minutes and are used before meals to control postprandial glucose levels. Regular insulin is an example of a short-acting insulin.

3. **Intermediate-Acting Insulin:** Intermediate-acting insulins have a more extended duration of action and are often used to provide basal insulin coverage. NPH insulin is a common intermediate-acting insulin.

4. **Long-Acting Insulin:** Long-acting insulins provide a steady release of insulin over an extended period, offering basal insulin coverage. Examples include insulin glargine and insulin detemir.

5. **Combination Insulin:** Some insulin formulations combine rapid-acting or short-acting insulin with intermediate-acting or long-acting insulin to provide both mealtime and basal coverage.

Inhaled Insulin: An Alternative Delivery Method

In recent years, inhaled insulin has emerged as an alternative delivery method for mealtime insulin. It is administered using an inhaler device and offers a non-invasive option for individuals who may prefer not to inject insulin. Inhaled insulin is a rapid-acting insulin and is typically used before meals.

Choosing the right medication or combination of medications depends on various factors, including the individual's overall health, lifestyle, and treatment goals. Healthcare providers work closely with individuals to tailor medication regimens, considering factors such as potential side effects, convenience, and adherence to the prescribed treatment plan.

Insulin Therapy: Types, Administration, and Dosage

Insulin therapy is a crucial component of diabetes management, particularly for individuals with Type 1 diabetes and some with Type 2 diabetes. Understanding the types of insulin, proper administration techniques, and dosage adjustments are essential for effective insulin therapy.

Types of Insulin: Matching Needs with Formulations

There are several types of insulin, each with its onset, peak, and duration of action. The main categories of insulin include:

1. **Rapid-Acting Insulin:** As the name suggests, rapid-acting insulin works quickly to lower blood sugar levels. It typically starts working within 15 minutes, peaks in about an hour, and lasts for 2 to 4 hours. Examples include insulin lispro, insulin aspart, and insulin glulisine.

2. **Short-Acting Insulin:** Short-acting insulin has a slightly slower onset compared to rapid-acting insulin. It starts working within 30 minutes, peaks in 2 to 3 hours, and lasts for around 3 to 6 hours. Regular insulin is an example of short-acting insulin.

3. **Intermediate-Acting Insulin:** Intermediate-acting insulin has a more extended duration of action, providing basal insulin coverage. It typically starts working within 2 to 4 hours, peaks in 4 to 12 hours, and lasts for up to 18 hours. NPH insulin is a common intermediate-acting insulin.

4. **Long-Acting Insulin:** Long-acting insulin provides a steady release of insulin over an extended period, offering basal insulin coverage. It has a gradual onset, peaks minimally, and lasts for up to 24 hours. Examples include insulin glargine and insulin detemir.

5. **Ultra-Long-Acting Insulin:** The newest category of insulin, ultra-long-acting insulin, has an even more extended duration of action, often exceeding 24 hours. Insulin degludec is an example of ultra-long-acting insulin.

Insulin Administration: Mastering the Techniques

Administering insulin involves more than just injecting the hormone. Proper technique ensures effective absorption and optimal blood sugar control. Here are key aspects of insulin administration:

1. **Subcutaneous Injection:** Insulin is typically injected into the subcutaneous tissue, the fatty layer just below the skin. Common injection sites include the abdomen, thighs, and upper arms.

2. **Rotating Injection Sites:** Regularly rotating injection sites help prevent the development of lumps or fatty deposits at the injection site, ensuring consistent insulin absorption.

3. **Injection Angle and Depth:** The angle and depth of the injection can impact insulin absorption. Healthcare providers provide guidance on the appropriate technique based on the type of insulin and individual factors.

4. **Proper Needle Size:** Using the correct needle size is crucial for comfortable and effective injections. Shorter needles are often suitable for subcutaneous injections, while longer needles may be required for individuals with thicker subcutaneous tissue.

5. **Injection Timing:** Administering insulin at consistent times each day helps maintain stable blood sugar levels. Timing

may vary depending on the type of insulin and individual lifestyle.

6. **Insulin Pens and Syringes:** Insulin pens and syringes are common tools for insulin administration. Pens offer convenience and premeasured doses, while syringes provide flexibility in adjusting doses.

Dosage Adjustments: Fine-Tuning Insulin Therapy

Achieving optimal blood sugar control often involves fine-tuning insulin dosages based on factors such as diet, physical activity, and overall health. Dosage adjustments may be necessary to address fluctuations in blood sugar levels and prevent hypoglycemia or hyperglycemia.

1. **Basal Insulin Adjustments:** Basal insulin provides a continuous release of insulin to control fasting blood sugar levels. Adjustments to basal insulin doses may be made to address changes in routine, such as meal timing or exercise.

2. **Bolus Insulin Adjustments:** Bolus insulin is administered before meals to cover the rise in blood sugar levels associated with eating. Adjustments may be needed based on the carbohydrate content of meals and individual insulin sensitivity.

3. **Correction Doses:** Correction doses, also known as supplemental or correctional insulin, may be prescribed to address unexpected high blood sugar levels. The dose is calculated based on the difference between the current blood sugar level and the target level.

4. **Regular Monitoring:** Regular blood glucose monitoring is essential for assessing the effectiveness of insulin therapy and identifying patterns that may require dosage adjustments. Individuals and healthcare providers work

collaboratively to make informed decisions about insulin dosages.

Understanding the nuances of insulin therapy empowers individuals to take an active role in their diabetes management. Open communication with healthcare providers, regular monitoring, and adherence to prescribed insulin regimens contribute to successful and personalized insulin therapy.

Chapter 3: Creating a Diabetes-Friendly Meal Plan

A diabetes-friendly meal plan is a crucial tool for managing blood sugar levels and promoting overall health. By making thoughtful food choices and incorporating nutrient-rich ingredients, individuals with diabetes can enjoy satisfying and balanced meals while supporting their well-being. In this chapter, we will explore the principles of creating a diabetes-friendly meal plan.

Understanding the Basics of a Diabetes-Friendly Meal Plan

Before delving into the specifics of superfoods and nutrient-rich ingredients, it's essential to understand the fundamental principles of a diabetes-friendly meal plan. The primary goals of such a plan are to regulate blood sugar levels, maintain a healthy weight, and reduce the risk of complications associated with diabetes.

1. **Balanced Carbohydrates:** Carbohydrates significantly impact blood sugar levels, making it crucial to choose complex carbohydrates that provide sustained energy. Include whole grains, legumes, and vegetables while moderating the intake of refined carbohydrates.

2. **Moderate Protein Intake:** Protein plays a role in satiety and muscle health. Include lean protein sources such as poultry, fish, tofu, legumes, and low-fat dairy products in your meals.

3. **Healthy Fats:** Opt for heart-healthy fats, such as those found in avocados, nuts, seeds, and olive oil. Limit saturated and trans fats, commonly found in fried foods and processed snacks.

4. **Portion Control:** Monitoring portion sizes helps manage calorie intake and prevents overeating. Pay attention to

recommended serving sizes and listen to your body's hunger and fullness cues.

5. **Fiber-rich foods:** High-fiber foods contribute to better blood sugar control and help with weight management. Incorporate fruits, vegetables, whole grains, and legumes to increase your fiber intake.

6. **Consistent Meal Timing:** Maintaining regular meal timing can help stabilize blood sugar levels. Aim for a consistent schedule with evenly spaced meals and snacks.

Understanding Carbohydrates, Proteins, and Fats in Diabetes

Creating a diabetes-friendly meal plan starts with a fundamental understanding of the macronutrients that make up our diet: carbohydrates, proteins, and fats. Each of these macronutrients plays a unique role in our body, and managing their intake is crucial for individuals with diabetes.

Carbohydrates: Balancing the Glucose Impact

Carbohydrates are the body's primary source of energy, and they directly impact blood sugar levels. When consumed, carbohydrates are broken down into glucose, raising blood sugar. For individuals with diabetes, understanding the type and quantity of carbohydrates is essential for managing blood sugar levels.

1. **Types of Carbohydrates:** Carbohydrates come in two main types—simple and complex. Simple carbohydrates, found in sugary foods and refined grains, are quickly digested and can cause rapid spikes in blood sugar. Complex carbohydrates, present in whole grains, fruits, and vegetables, are digested more slowly, leading to a gradual and steady increase in blood sugar.

2. **Glycemic Index (GI):** The glycemic index measures how quickly a carbohydrate-containing food raises blood sugar. Foods with a high GI cause a rapid spike, while those with a low GI result in a slower and more controlled increase. Choosing lower GI foods can help regulate blood sugar levels more effectively.

3. **Carb Counting:** Carb counting involves monitoring the number of carbohydrates consumed in a meal. This method helps individuals with diabetes manage their insulin doses more accurately and maintain better control over blood sugar levels.

4. **Fiber: A Carb with Benefits:** Fiber is a type of carbohydrate that is not fully digested. High-fiber foods, such as whole grains, legumes, fruits, and vegetables, provide numerous health benefits. Fiber slows down the digestion of carbohydrates, leading to a more gradual release of glucose into the bloodstream.

Proteins: Building Blocks for Health

Proteins play a crucial role in the body, serving as building blocks for tissues, muscles, enzymes, and hormones. Including an adequate amount of protein in a diabetes-friendly meal plan can contribute to satiety and help manage blood sugar levels.

1. **Lean Protein Sources:** Opt for lean protein sources to reduce saturated fat intake. Examples of lean proteins include poultry, fish, tofu, legumes, and low-fat dairy products. These choices provide essential nutrients without contributing excessive calories or unhealthy fats.

2. **Portion Control:** While protein is an essential part of a balanced diet, it's crucial not to overconsume. Practicing portion control helps maintain a balanced and varied meal plan. Aiming for a palm-sized portion of protein per meal is a general guideline.

3. **Plant-Based Proteins:** Plant-based proteins, such as beans, lentils, quinoa, and nuts, offer an excellent alternative for those looking to incorporate more plant-based options into their meal plans. These protein sources also provide additional nutrients and fiber.

4. **Timing Matters:** Distributing protein intake throughout the day can contribute to better blood sugar management. Including protein in each meal and snack helps stabilize blood sugar levels and promotes a feeling of fullness.

Fats: Choosing Wisely for Heart Health

While fats have been traditionally viewed with caution, they are an essential component of a healthy diet. However, the type of fats consumed matters, especially for individuals with diabetes who are at a higher risk of heart disease.

1. **Healthy Fats:** Focus on incorporating healthy fats into the meal plan. These include monounsaturated fats found in olive oil, avocados, and nuts, as well as polyunsaturated fats present in fatty fish, flaxseeds, and walnuts. These fats contribute to heart health and overall well-being.

2. **Limit Saturated and Trans Fats:** Saturated and trans fats, often found in processed and fried foods, can raise cholesterol levels and contribute to heart disease. Limiting the intake of foods high in these fats is essential for cardiovascular health.

3. **Balancing Omega-3 and Omega-6 Fatty Acids:** Omega-3 fatty acids, found in fatty fish like salmon and trout, as well as flaxseeds and chia seeds, have anti-inflammatory properties and benefit heart health. Balancing the ratio of omega-3 to omega-6 fatty acids is crucial for overall well-being.

4. **Mindful Cooking Methods:** Choosing healthier cooking methods, such as baking, grilling, steaming, or sautéing,

helps minimize the use of added fats and promotes the retention of nutrients in the food.

Understanding the role of carbohydrates, proteins, and fats in the context of diabetes empowers individuals to make informed choices that support both blood sugar management and overall health. The key is to strike a balance and choose nutrient-dense foods that provide essential vitamins, minerals, and energy without causing drastic spikes in blood sugar.

Meal Planning Strategies for Balanced Nutrition

Creating a diabetes-friendly meal plan is a fundamental aspect of managing blood sugar levels and promoting overall health. A well-balanced and nutritious diet plays a crucial role in diabetes management, providing essential nutrients while helping to regulate glucose levels. In this section, we will explore effective meal-planning strategies tailored for individuals living with diabetes.

Understanding Carbohydrate Counting: The Foundation of Diabetes Meal Planning

Carbohydrate counting is a key strategy in diabetes meal planning, as carbohydrates have a direct impact on blood sugar levels. Carbohydrates are broken down into glucose during digestion, leading to an increase in blood sugar. By understanding and managing carbohydrate intake, individuals can better control their blood glucose levels.

1. **Identifying Carbohydrate Sources:** Knowing which foods contain carbohydrates is the first step in effective carbohydrate counting. Common sources include grains, fruits, vegetables, legumes, dairy products, and sweets.

2. **Portion Control:** Managing portion sizes is crucial for carbohydrate counting. Measuring food portions or using visual cues can help individuals consume appropriate amounts of carbohydrates without causing significant spikes in blood sugar.

3. **Glycemic Index Consideration:** The glycemic index (GI) measures how quickly a food raises blood sugar levels. Foods with a high GI can cause rapid spikes, while those with a low GI lead to slower, more gradual increases. Choosing lower GI foods can be beneficial in maintaining stable blood glucose levels.

4. **Balancing Macronutrients:** In addition to carbohydrates, it's essential to consider protein and fats in meal planning. Including a balance of macronutrients helps stabilize blood sugar levels, promote satiety, and provide sustained energy.

The Plate Method: Simplifying Portion Control

The plate method is a visual and straightforward approach to meal planning that helps control portion sizes and balance macronutrients. It involves dividing the plate into three sections:

1. **Half the Plate for Non-Starchy Vegetables:** Non-starchy vegetables, such as leafy greens, broccoli, cauliflower, and peppers, fill half the plate. These vegetables are low in carbohydrates and rich in fiber, vitamins, and minerals.

2. **One-Quarter of the Plate for Lean Proteins:** Protein is an essential component of a diabetes-friendly meal plan. Lean protein sources, such as poultry, fish, tofu, or legumes, occupy one-quarter of the plate. Protein helps stabilize blood sugar levels and supports muscle health.

3. **One-Quarter of the Plate for Whole Grains or Starchy Vegetables:** The remaining quarter of the plate is dedicated to whole grains or starchy vegetables. Opting for whole grains like brown rice, quinoa, or sweet potatoes provides complex carbohydrates, fiber, and additional nutrients.

Fiber-Rich Foods: Promoting Satiety and Blood Sugar Control

Including fiber-rich foods in a diabetes-friendly meal plan offers numerous benefits. Fiber slows down the digestion and absorption of carbohydrates, leading to more stable blood sugar levels. Additionally, high-fiber foods contribute to a feeling of fullness and can aid in weight management. Key sources of dietary fiber include:

1. **Whole Grains:** Choose whole grains like oats, barley, quinoa, and whole wheat over refined grains. These grains contain more fiber and nutrients, promoting better blood sugar control.

2. **Legumes:** Beans, lentils, and chickpeas are excellent sources of fiber and protein. Adding legumes to meals provides a sustained release of energy and helps regulate blood sugar levels.

3. **Vegetables and Fruits:** Non-starchy vegetables and certain fruits, such as berries and apples, are rich in fiber. Including a variety of colorful fruits and vegetables in the diet adds nutritional diversity and supports overall well-being.

4. **Nuts and Seeds:** Nuts and seeds, such as almonds, chia seeds, and flaxseeds, are packed with fiber, healthy fats, and essential nutrients. They make for nutritious snacks or additions to meals.

Regular Meal Timing and Consistency: Stabilizing Blood Sugar Levels

Consistency in meal timing is crucial for individuals with diabetes to help regulate blood sugar levels and prevent extreme fluctuations. A routine with regular meals and snacks throughout the day provides a steady supply of nutrients and energy. Key considerations for meal timing include:

1. **Eating at Regular Intervals:** Spacing meals evenly throughout the day helps avoid prolonged periods without food, preventing drops or spikes in blood sugar levels.

2. **Including Snacks as Needed:** Healthy snacks can be incorporated between meals to maintain steady energy

levels and prevent overeating during main meals. Opt for snacks that combine protein and fiber for sustained satiety.

3. **Avoiding Skipping Meals:** Skipping meals can lead to irregular blood sugar levels. Consistent meal patterns contribute to better glycemic control and overall well-being.

4. **Monitoring Blood Sugar Responses:** Monitoring blood sugar levels before and after meals provides valuable insights into how specific foods and meal combinations impact individual responses. This information can guide adjustments to the meal plan for better blood sugar control.

Individualized Meal Planning: Tailoring Strategies to Personal Preferences and Health Goals

Creating a diabetes-friendly meal plan is not a one-size-fits-all approach. It requires consideration of individual preferences, cultural influences, and health goals. Tailoring the meal plan to align with personal tastes and lifestyle factors increases adherence and enhances the overall quality of life.

1. **Cultural Considerations:** Recognizing and respecting cultural preferences is essential in developing a sustainable and enjoyable meal plan. Integrating familiar foods while making mindful choices helps individuals embrace a diabetes-friendly diet without sacrificing cultural identity.

2. **Personal Preferences:** Considering individual likes and dislikes ensures that the meal plan is both enjoyable and satisfying. Exploring new recipes, flavors, and cooking techniques can add variety to the diet and keep meals interesting.

3. **Health Goals and Restrictions:** Understanding specific health goals, such as weight management or cholesterol control, allows for targeted meal planning. Individuals with diabetes may also have other health conditions that require dietary

modifications, and these considerations should be incorporated into the meal plan.

4. **Flexible Approaches:** Recognizing that life events, social occasions, or unexpected circumstances may impact meal planning allows for a flexible approach. Providing guidelines rather than rigid rules fosters adaptability and long-term success.

Incorporating these meal planning strategies into daily life empowers individuals with diabetes to take control of their nutrition, support overall health, and maintain stable blood sugar levels. The key is to strike a balance between enjoyment, variety, and mindful choices while considering individual needs and preferences.

Incorporating Superfoods and Nutrient-Rich Ingredients

Superfoods and nutrient-rich ingredients are powerhouse foods that offer a multitude of health benefits. Incorporating these into a diabetes-friendly meal plan can enhance nutritional value while adding variety and flavor. Let's explore how to integrate these ingredients into different aspects of your meals:

Breakfast: Energizing Start to the Day

1. **Chia Seeds: A Fiber Boost:** Chia seeds are rich in soluble fiber, which can help stabilize blood sugar levels. Add a tablespoon of chia seeds to your breakfast yogurt or smoothie for an extra fiber boost.

2. **Berries: Antioxidant Powerhouse:** Berries like blueberries, strawberries, and raspberries are packed with antioxidants, vitamins, and fiber. Enjoy them on top of oatmeal or mixed into a bowl of Greek yogurt for a delicious and nutritious start to your day.

3. **Quinoa: Protein-Packed Grain:** Quinoa is a complete protein source, making it an excellent choice for breakfast. Prepare a

quinoa bowl with fresh fruit, nuts, and a drizzle of honey for a protein-packed and satisfying morning meal.

Lunch: Nourishing and Satisfying

1. **Leafy Greens: Nutrient-Rich Foundation:** Leafy greens like spinach, kale, and Swiss chard are rich in vitamins, minerals, and antioxidants. Use them as the base for your lunch salads or add them to wraps and sandwiches for a nutrient-packed lunch.

2. **Salmon: Omega-3 Goodness:** Fatty fish like salmon are high in omega-3 fatty acids, which have anti-inflammatory properties. Grill or bake salmon and pair it with a colorful salad for a delicious and diabetes-friendly lunch.

3. **Quinoa Salad: Fiber and Protein Combo:** Create a quinoa salad with a variety of colorful vegetables, such as bell peppers, cherry tomatoes, and cucumbers. The combination of quinoa and vegetables provides a satisfying mix of fiber and protein.

Dinner: Balanced and Flavorful

1. **Sweet Potatoes: Complex Carbohydrate Source:** Sweet potatoes are a nutrient-rich alternative to regular potatoes. Roast or mash sweet potatoes as a side dish for your dinner. They provide complex carbohydrates, fiber, and vitamins.

2. **Broccoli: Fiber and Antioxidants:** Broccoli is a cruciferous vegetable rich in fiber and antioxidants. Include steamed or roasted broccoli as a side dish to add nutritional value and vibrant flavor to your dinner plate.

3. **Tofu: Plant-Based Protein Option:** Tofu is a versatile plant-based protein source. Incorporate tofu into stir-fries, curries, or grilled dishes for a satisfying and diabetes-friendly dinner.

Snacks: Healthy and Satisfying Options

1. **Almonds: Nutrient-Dense Snacking:** Almonds are a nutrient-dense snack rich in healthy fats, protein, and fiber. Enjoy a handful of almonds as a satisfying and blood-sugar-friendly snack between meals.

2. **Greek Yogurt: Protein-Packed Delight:** Greek yogurt is a protein-packed snack that also provides probiotics for gut health. Add a sprinkle of berries or a drizzle of honey for extra flavor and nutrients.

3. **Edamame: Plant-Based Protein Bite:** Edamame, or young soybeans, are a tasty and protein-rich snack. Steam or boil edamame and lightly season with salt for a satisfying and diabetes-friendly nibble.

Desserts: Sweet Indulgences in Moderation

1. **Dark Chocolate: Antioxidant-Rich Treat:** Dark chocolate with high cocoa content is rich in antioxidants and may have benefits for heart health. Enjoy a small piece as an occasional dessert, keeping portion sizes in mind.

2. **Baked Apples: Naturally Sweet Delight:** Baked apples with a sprinkle of cinnamon make for a naturally sweet and diabetes-friendly dessert. The fiber in apples helps slow down the absorption of sugars.

3. **Yogurt Parfait: Balanced Sweetness:** Create a yogurt parfait with layers of Greek yogurt, fresh berries, and a small amount of granola. This dessert provides a balance of sweetness, protein, and fiber.

Tips for Successful Meal Planning

1. **Diversify Your Plate:** Aim for a colorful and diverse plate with a variety of vegetables, lean proteins, and whole grains. This ensures a mix of essential nutrients.

2. **Mindful Eating:** Practice mindful eating by savoring each bite, paying attention to hunger and fullness cues, and avoiding distractions during meals.

3. **Hydration:** Stay well-hydrated by drinking water throughout the day. Limit sugary drinks and opt for water, herbal tea, or infused water for added flavor.

4. **Meal Timing:** Space your meals and snacks evenly throughout the day to help regulate blood sugar levels. Avoid skipping meals, as this can lead to overeating later in the day.

5. **Consult with a Dietitian:** If possible, consult with a registered dietitian or nutritionist specializing in diabetes care. They can provide personalized guidance based on your health status, preferences, and lifestyle.

Incorporating superfoods and nutrient-rich ingredients into your diabetes-friendly meal plan not only supports blood sugar management but also contributes to overall well-being. Experiment with different recipes, flavors, and combinations to discover a variety of delicious and nutritious options that fit your dietary preferences and health goals. Remember, creating a sustainable and enjoyable meal plan is an ongoing process of exploration and adaptation.

Chapter 4. Diabetes-Friendly Recipes and Food Types

Sample Diabetes-Friendly Recipes

Recipe 1: Quinoa and Vegetable Buddha Bowl

Ingredients:

- 1 cup cooked quinoa

- 1 cup broccoli florets

- 1 cup cherry tomatoes, halved

- 1 cup sliced bell peppers (assorted colors)

- 1/2 cup shredded carrots

- 1/4 cup sliced cucumber

- 2 tablespoons olive oil

- 1 tablespoon balsamic vinegar

- 1 teaspoon Dijon mustard

- Salt and pepper to taste

- 1/4 cup crumbled feta cheese (optional)

- Fresh herbs for garnish (parsley or cilantro)

Instructions:

1. In a large bowl, combine the cooked quinoa, broccoli, cherry tomatoes, bell peppers, shredded carrots, and sliced cucumber.

2. In a small bowl, whisk together olive oil, balsamic vinegar, Dijon mustard, salt, and pepper to create the dressing.

3. Pour the dressing over the quinoa and vegetables, tossing gently to coat everything evenly.

4. Divide the mixture into serving bowls.

5. If desired, top each bowl with crumbled feta cheese and fresh herbs for added flavor.

6. Serve immediately and enjoy your nutrient-packed Quinoa and Vegetable Buddha Bowl!

Recipe 2: Grilled Salmon with Lemon-Dill Sauce

Ingredients:

- 4 salmon fillets

- 2 tablespoons olive oil

- 1 teaspoon dried dill

- 1 teaspoon garlic powder

- Salt and pepper to taste

- Lemon wedges for serving

For the Lemon-Dill Sauce:

- 1/2 cup Greek yogurt

- 1 tablespoon fresh dill, finely chopped

- 1 tablespoon lemon juice

- Zest of one lemon

- Salt and pepper to taste

Instructions:

1. Preheat the grill to medium-high heat.

2. In a small bowl, mix olive oil, dried dill, garlic powder, salt, and pepper. Brush the mixture over the salmon fillets.

3. Place the salmon fillets on the preheated grill and cook for 4-5 minutes per side, or until the salmon is cooked through and easily flakes with a fork.

4. While the salmon is grilling, prepare the Lemon-Dill Sauce. In a bowl, combine Greek yogurt, fresh dill, lemon juice, lemon zest, salt, and pepper. Mix well.

5. Once the salmon is done, transfer it to serving plates, and drizzle with the Lemon-Dill Sauce.

6. Serve the grilled salmon with lemon wedges on the side for an extra burst of citrus flavor.

7. Enjoy a delightful and protein-rich Grilled Salmon with Lemon-Dill Sauce!

Recipe 3: Cauliflower Fried Rice with Tofu

Ingredients:

- 1 medium head of cauliflower, grated (or cauliflower rice)

- 1 cup firm tofu, cubed

- 1 cup mixed vegetables (peas, carrots, corn)

- 1/2 cup chopped green onions

- 2 cloves garlic, minced

- 2 tablespoons low-sodium soy sauce

- 1 tablespoon sesame oil

- 1 tablespoon olive oil

- 1 teaspoon ginger, grated

- Salt and pepper to taste

- Sesame seeds for garnish

Instructions:

1. In a large skillet, heat olive oil over medium heat. Add cubed tofu and cook until golden brown on all sides. Remove tofu from the skillet and set aside.

2. In the same skillet, add minced garlic and grated ginger. Sauté for 1-2 minutes until fragrant.

3. Add the mixed vegetables to the skillet and stir-fry until they are tender-crisp.

4. Push the vegetables to the side of the skillet and add cauliflower rice. Cook for 3-4 minutes, stirring occasionally.

5. Combine the cooked tofu with the vegetables and cauliflower rice. Mix well.

6. In a small bowl, whisk together soy sauce and sesame oil. Pour the sauce over the cauliflower mixture, tossing to coat evenly.

7. Season with salt and pepper to taste. Stir in chopped green onions.

8. Continue cooking for an additional 2-3 minutes until everything is heated through.

9. Garnish with sesame seeds before serving.

10. Serve this delicious Cauliflower Fried Rice with Tofu as a satisfying and low-carb alternative to traditional fried rice.

These diabetes-friendly recipes are designed to be flavorful, nutritious, and suitable for managing blood sugar levels. Experiment with these dishes and feel free to customize them according to your taste preferences and dietary needs. Remember to consult with your healthcare provider or a registered dietitian for personalized advice on your diabetes management journey.

Diabetes-Friendly Food Types

Non-Starchy Vegetables

Here is a table featuring non-starchy vegetable foods suitable for adults living with diabetes:

Food Type	Portion Size	Low Glycemic Index (GI)	Nutritional Information
Spinach	1 cup raw	Low	Rich in iron, vitamins A and K, and a good source of fiber
Broccoli	1 cup raw	Low	High in vitamin C, fiber, and various antioxidants
Cauliflower	1 cup raw	Low	Packed with vitamin C, and fiber, and is a versatile cooking option
Bell Peppers	1 medium	Low	Excellent source of vitamin C and various antioxidants
Zucchini	1 medium	Low	Low-calorie option with a good dose of vitamins and minerals
Cucumber	1 cup sliced	Low	Hydrating, low-calorie choice with vitamins and minerals
Asparagus	1 cup raw	Low	Rich in folate, and vitamin K, and a good source of fiber

Food Type	Portion Size	Low Glycemic Index (GI)	Nutritional Information
Brussels Sprouts	1 cup raw	Low	High in fiber, vitamins C and K, and antioxidants
Green Beans	1 cup raw	Low	Good source of vitamins C and K, plus folate
Kale	1 cup raw	Low	Nutrient-dense, with high amounts of vitamins A, C, and K
Artichokes	1 medium	Low	High in fiber, antioxidants, and vitamin C
Cabbage	1 cup shredded	Low	Low-calorie, rich in vitamin C and K, with potential anti-inflammatory benefits
Eggplant	1 cup cooked	Low	Low-calorie provides dietary fiber and various nutrients
Mushrooms	1 cup raw	Low	Low in carbs, high in selenium, and a good source of B vitamins
Radishes	1 cup sliced	Low	Low in calories, a good source of vitamin C
Celery	1 stalk	Low	Low-calorie, hydrating, and contains some fiber

Food Type	Portion Size	Low Glycemic Index (GI)	Nutritional Information
Tomatoes	1 medium	Low	Rich in vitamin C, potassium, and the antioxidant lycopene
Onions	1 medium	Low	Good source of vitamin C, fiber, and antioxidants
Carrots	1 medium	Moderate	High in beta-carotene, fiber, and vitamin K
Sugar Snap Peas	1 cup raw	Low	Crunchy and sweet, low-calorie, and a source of vitamin C

Keep in mind that individual responses to food can vary, and it's essential to monitor blood sugar levels and consult with a healthcare professional or a registered dietitian for personalized dietary advice.

WHOLE-FRUITS

Food Type	Portion Size	Low Glycemic Index (GI)	Nutritional Information
Berries (e.g., blueberries, strawberries)	1 cup	Low	Rich in antioxidants, vitamins C and K, and fiber

Food Type	Portion Size	Low Glycemic Index (GI)	Nutritional Information
Apples	1 medium	Low	Good source of fiber, vitamin C, and various antioxidants
Pears	1 medium	Low	High in dietary fiber, vitamins C and K
Oranges	1 medium	Low	Excellent source of vitamin C, fiber, and immune-boosting nutrients
Grapefruit	1/2 medium	Low	Low in calories, high in vitamin C and fiber
Kiwi	1 medium	Low	Rich in vitamin C, vitamin K, and dietary fiber
Peaches	1 medium	Low	Low-calorie, good source of vitamins A and C
Plums	2 medium	Low	Rich in antioxidants, vitamins K and A, and fiber
Cherries	1 cup	Low	Contains antioxidants, including anthocyanins, and vitamin C
Mango	1 cup sliced	Moderate	Provides vitamin C, and vitamin A, and is a good source of natural sugars

Food Type	Portion Size	Low Glycemic Index (GI)	Nutritional Information
Pineapple	1 cup chunks	Moderate	Contains bromelain, vitamin C, and manganese
Bananas	1 medium	Moderate	Good source of potassium, vitamin C, and dietary fiber
Watermelon	1 cup cubes	High	Hydrating, low-calorie, and contains vitamins A and C
Cantaloupe	1 cup cubes	Low	Rich in vitamins A and C, and a good source of hydration
Grapes	1 cup	Moderate	Contain antioxidants, such as resveratrol, and vitamin C
Strawberries	1 cup	Low	Low in calories, high in vitamin C, and antioxidants
Papaya	1 cup cubes	Low	High in vitamin C, and vitamin A, and contains the enzyme papain
Cranberries	1 cup	Low	Rich in antioxidants and vitamin C, known for urinary health benefits

Food Type	Portion Size	Low Glycemic Index (GI)	Nutritional Information
Apricots	3 medium	Low	Good source of vitamin A, vitamin C, and dietary fiber
Raspberries	1 cup	Low	High in fiber, vitamin C, and antioxidants
Blackberries	1 cup	Low	Rich in fiber, vitamin C, and antioxidants
Nectarines	1 medium	Low	Low-calorie, good source of vitamins A and C
Figs	4 medium	Low	Provide fiber, vitamins A and K, and natural sweetness
Guava	1 medium	Low	High in dietary fiber, vitamin C, and antioxidants
Avocado	1 medium	Low	Contains healthy monounsaturated fats, vitamins K, C, and E
Lemon	1 medium	Low	Low-calorie, high in vitamin C, and aids digestion
Lime	1 medium	Low	Low in calories, high in vitamin C, and adds a tangy flavor

Food Type	Portion Size	Low Glycemic Index (GI)	Nutritional Information
Passion Fruit	1 medium	Low	Low in calories, rich in fiber, and provides vitamin C
Kiwifruit	1 medium	Low	High in vitamin C, vitamin K, and dietary fiber
Tangerines	1 medium	Low	Good source of vitamin C, fiber, and natural sweetness
Dragon Fruit	1 cup cubes	Low	Low-calorie, high in vitamin C, and contains beneficial antioxidants

It's important to consider individual responses to fruits, monitor blood sugar levels, and consult with healthcare professionals or dietitians for personalized dietary advice.

LEAN PROTEINS

Here's a table featuring lean protein foods suitable for adults living with diabetes:

Food Type	Portion Size	Low Glycemic Index (GI)	Nutritional Information
Chicken Breast	3 oz cooked	N/A (Low)	High in protein, low in fat, a good source of B vitamins and minerals

Food Type	Portion Size	Low Glycemic Index (GI)	Nutritional Information
Turkey Breast	3 oz cooked	N/A (Low)	Lean protein, low in saturated fat, provides vitamins and minerals
Salmon	3 oz cooked	N/A (Low)	Rich in omega-3 fatty acids, high-quality protein, and vitamin D
Tuna	3 oz canned	N/A (Low)	Low in calories, high in protein, a good source of omega-3 fatty acids
Cod	3 oz cooked	N/A (Low)	Lean white fish, low in fat, high in protein
Shrimp	3 oz cooked	N/A (Low)	Low in calories, high in protein, a good source of selenium
Eggs	2 large	N/A (Low)	Excellent source of protein, vitamins B12, D, and essential minerals
Lean Ground Beef	3 oz cooked	N/A (Low)	Provides protein, iron, zinc, and other essential nutrients
Greek Yogurt	6 oz	N/A (Low)	High in protein, probiotics, and calcium
Cottage Cheese	1 cup	N/A (Low)	Rich in protein, low in carbohydrates, a source of calcium

Food Type	Portion Size	Low Glycemic Index (GI)	Nutritional Information
Tofu	3 oz cooked	N/A (Low)	Plant-based protein, low in saturated fat, and a good source of iron
Lentils	1 cup cooked	Low	Plant-based protein, high in fiber, and provides essential nutrients
Chickpeas	1 cup cooked	Low	Good source of plant-based protein, fiber, and vitamins
Quinoa	1 cup cooked	Low	Complete protein, high in fiber, and contains essential amino acids
Lean Pork Tenderloin	3 oz cooked	N/A (Low)	Low in fat, high in protein, provides B vitamins and zinc
Skinless Turkey Sausage	3 oz cooked	N/A (Low)	Lean protein option with fewer saturated fats
Low-Fat Cottage Cheese	1 cup	N/A (Low)	High in protein, low in fat, and a source of calcium
Swordfish	3 oz cooked	N/A (Low)	High-quality protein, rich in omega-3 fatty acids
Greek Chicken Souvlaki	1 skewer	N/A (Low)	Grilled chicken with herbs, providing protein and Mediterranean flavors

Food Type	Portion Size	Low Glycemic Index (GI)	Nutritional Information
Mackerel	3 oz cooked	N/A (Low)	Fatty fish rich in omega-3s, high-quality protein
Skim Milk	1 cup	N/A (Low)	Good source of protein, calcium, and vitamin D
Edamame	1 cup	N/A (Low)	Plant-based protein, high in fiber, and provides essential nutrients
Bison	3 oz cooked	N/A (Low)	Lean protein option, lower in fat compared to beef
Greek Salad with Feta	1 serving	N/A (Low)	Includes chicken, feta, and vegetables for a balanced meal
Walnuts	1 oz	N/A (Low)	Plant-based protein, omega-3 fatty acids, and essential nutrients
Tempeh	3 oz cooked	N/A (Low)	Fermented soy product, rich in protein and nutrients
Seitan	3 oz cooked	N/A (Low)	High-protein meat substitute made from gluten
Chicken Stir-Fry	1 serving	N/A (Low)	Includes lean chicken, assorted vegetables, and a light sauce

Food Type	Portion Size	Low Glycemic Index (GI)	Nutritional Information
Ground Chicken	3 oz cooked	N/A (Low)	Lean protein option, versatile for various recipes
Almonds	1 oz	N/A (Low)	Plant-based protein, healthy fats, and a good source of vitamins
Pinto Beans	1 cup cooked	Low	Plant-based protein, high in fiber, and provides essential nutrients

Remember to consider individual dietary needs, monitor blood sugar levels, and consult with healthcare professionals or dietitians for personalized dietary advice.

WHOLE GRAINS

Here's a table featuring whole-grain foods suitable for adults living with diabetes:

Food Type	Portion Size	Low Glycemic Index (GI)	Nutritional Information
Brown Rice	1 cup cooked	Medium	High in fiber, vitamins, and minerals, a good source of complex carbs

Food Type	Portion Size	Low Glycemic Index (GI)	Nutritional Information
Quinoa	1 cup cooked	Low	Complete protein, high in fiber, and contains essential amino acids
Oats	1/2 cup dry	Low	Rich in soluble fiber, helps with blood sugar control and heart health
Barley	1 cup cooked	Medium	High in fiber, vitamins, and minerals, supports heart health
Bulgur	1 cup cooked	Low	Low-calorie, high in fiber, and provides essential nutrients
Whole Wheat Bread	1 slice	Low	Good source of fiber, vitamins, and minerals
Whole Wheat Pasta	1 cup cooked	Low	Higher fiber content compared to traditional pasta
Farro	1 cup cooked	Low	Nutrient-dense whole grain, high in fiber, and rich in antioxidants
Freekeh	1 cup cooked	Low	High in fiber and protein, provides essential nutrients

Food Type	Portion Size	Low Glycemic Index (GI)	Nutritional Information
Buckwheat	1 cup cooked	Low	Gluten-free whole grain, rich in fiber, and provides essential nutrients
Millet	1 cup cooked	Low	Gluten-free, high in magnesium, and a good source of fiber
Amaranth	1 cup cooked	Low	Gluten-free, high in protein, and contains essential amino acids
Spelt	1 cup cooked	Low	Nutrient-dense whole grain provides fiber and various vitamins
Teff	1 cup cooked	Low	Gluten-free, rich in iron, calcium, and protein
Rye	1 slice	Low	Provides fiber, vitamins, and minerals, and supports digestive health
Sorghum	1 cup cooked	Low	Gluten-free, high in fiber, and provides essential nutrients
Whole Grain Tortillas	1 tortilla	Low	A good alternative for wraps, providing fiber and nutrients

Food Type	Portion Size	Low Glycemic Index (GI)	Nutritional Information
Whole Grain Crackers	10 crackers	Low	Whole grain option for snacks, providing fiber and some vitamins
Whole Grain Cereal	1 cup	Low	Choose options with minimal added sugars and high fiber content
Brown Rice Cakes	2 cakes	Low	Low-calorie snack can be topped with nut butter or veggies
Whole Wheat English Muffin	1 muffin	Low	High in fiber, makes for a nutritious breakfast or snack
Buckwheat Pancakes	2 pancakes	Low	Gluten-free option, rich in fiber and nutrients
Whole Grain Bagel	1 bagel	Low	Choose whole grain varieties for added fiber and nutrients
Whole Wheat Pita Bread	1 pita	Low	Great for sandwiches or wraps, provides fiber and complex carbs
Whole Wheat Pretzels	10 pretzels	Low	A low-fat snack option, choose those without excessive salt

Food Type	Portion Size	Low Glycemic Index (GI)	Nutritional Information
Brown Rice Noodles	1 cup cooked	Low	A gluten-free alternative to traditional noodles, high in fiber
Whole Grain Waffles	2 waffles	Low	Choose varieties with whole-grain ingredients for added nutrients
Whole Grain Muffins	1 muffin	Low	Homemade or store-bought, check for whole-grain ingredients
Whole Wheat Couscous	1 cup cooked	Low	A quick-cooking option, high in fiber and nutrients
Whole Grain Rice Crackers	15 crackers	Low	Snack option with a satisfying crunch, choose those with whole grains
Whole Wheat Flour	1/4 cup	Low	Use in baking for a healthier option, adds fiber to recipes
Whole Grain Pizza Crust	1 slice	Low	Make homemade pizzas with a whole-grain crust for added nutrition
Whole Wheat Pancake Mix	1 cup	Low	Choose mixes with whole grain ingredients, add fruits for extra flavor

Food Type	Portion Size	Low Glycemic Index (GI)	Nutritional Information
Whole Grain Granola	1/2 cup	Low	Opt for varieties with lower added sugars and higher fiber content
Whole Wheat Pretzel Twists	10 twists	Low	A crunchy snack option, choose those with whole grain ingredients
Whole Grain Rice Cereal	1 cup	Low	Fortified with vitamins and minerals, choose options with minimal sugar
Brown Rice Tortillas	1 tortilla	Low	Gluten-free alternative, suitable for wraps and tacos
Whole Grain Hot Cereal	1/2 cup dry	Low	Choose options with minimal added sugars, high in fiber
Whole Wheat Flatbread	1 piece	Low	Ideal for sandwiches or pizza, provides fiber and nutrients

When including whole grains in your diet, it's essential to monitor portion sizes and consider individual dietary needs. Consult with healthcare professionals or dietitians for personalized dietary advice.

HEALTHY FATS

Here's a table featuring healthy fat foods suitable for adults living with diabetes:

Food Type	Portion Size	Low Glycemic Index (GI)	Nutritional Information
Avocado	1/2 medium	Low	Rich in monounsaturated fats, fiber, vitamins, and minerals
Olive Oil	1 tablespoon	N/A (Low)	Heart-healthy monounsaturated fats, antioxidants, and vitamin E
Nuts (Almonds, Walnuts)	1 oz (handful)	N/A (Low)	Provides healthy fats, protein, and a variety of vitamins and minerals
Chia Seeds	2 tablespoons	Low	High in omega-3 fatty acids, fiber, and antioxidants
Flaxseeds	2 tablespoons	Low	Good source of omega-3 fatty acids, fiber, and lignans
Salmon	3 oz cooked	N/A (Low)	Rich in omega-3 fatty acids, high-quality protein, and vitamin D
Mackerel	3 oz cooked	N/A (Low)	Fatty fish rich in omega-3s, high-quality protein

Food Type	Portion Size	Low Glycemic Index (GI)	Nutritional Information
Walnuts	1 oz	N/A (Low)	Plant-based omega-3 fatty acids, antioxidants, and essential nutrients
Almonds	1 oz	N/A (Low)	Nutrient-dense, providing healthy fats, protein, and vitamins
Pecans	1 oz	N/A (Low)	Rich in monounsaturated fats, fiber, and essential minerals
Dark Chocolate (70% cocoa)	1 oz	Low	Contains antioxidants and may have heart health benefits
Sunflower Seeds	1 oz	N/A (Low)	Healthy fats, protein, vitamin E, and other essential nutrients
Olive Tapenade	2 tablespoons	N/A (Low)	Made with olives, capers, and olive oil, rich in healthy fats
Coconut Oil	1 tablespoon	Low	Contains medium-chain triglycerides (MCTs) and may support weight management
Avocado Oil	1 tablespoon	N/A (Low)	Rich in monounsaturated fats, vitamin E, and antioxidants

Food Type	Portion Size	Low Glycemic Index (GI)	Nutritional Information
Pumpkin Seeds	1 oz	N/A (Low)	Good source of healthy fats, protein, and magnesium
Cashews	1 oz	N/A (Low)	Provides healthy fats, protein, and important minerals
Hemp Seeds	2 tablespoons	Low	High in omega-3 and omega-6 fatty acids, protein, and fiber
Olive Tapenade	2 tablespoons	N/A (Low)	Made with olives, capers, and olive oil, rich in healthy fats
Edamame	1 cup	N/A (Low)	Plant-based protein, healthy fats, and a good source of fiber
Greek Yogurt (Full-fat)	1 cup	N/A (Low)	Provides healthy fats, protein, probiotics, and essential nutrients
Dark chocolate-covered almonds	1 oz	Low	Combines the benefits of almonds with the antioxidants in dark chocolate
Hummus	2 tablespoons	Low	Made from chickpeas and olive oil, provides healthy fats and protein

Food Type	Portion Size	Low Glycemic Index (GI)	Nutritional Information
Nut Butters (Almond, Peanut)	2 tablespoons	N/A (Low)	Good source of healthy fats, protein, and various vitamins and minerals
Tahini	1 tablespoon	N/A (Low)	Sesame seed paste, rich in healthy fats, protein, and minerals
Fatty Fish (Trout, Sardines)	3 oz cooked	N/A (Low)	Rich in omega-3 fatty acids, high-quality protein, and vitamin D
Coconut Milk	1 cup	N/A (Low)	Provides healthy fats and a creamy texture, suitable for cooking
Cheese (Feta, Goat)	1 oz	N/A (Low)	Contains healthy fats, protein, and essential nutrients
Pistachios	1 oz	N/A (Low)	Provides healthy fats, protein, and a variety of vitamins and minerals
Olives (Kalamata, Green)	1 oz	N/A (Low)	Low in carbs, high in healthy fats, and a source of antioxidants
Yogurt Parfait with Nuts	1 serving	N/A (Low)	Combines yogurt with nuts for a nutritious and satisfying snack

Food Type	Portion Size	Low Glycemic Index (GI)	Nutritional Information
Seaweed (Nori Sheets)	1 sheet	Low	Contains healthy fats, vitamins, and minerals
Almond Flour	1/4 cup	N/A (Low)	A gluten-free alternative for baking, high in healthy fats and protein
Guacamole	1/2 cup	Low	Avocado-based dip with healthy fats, fiber, and essential nutrients
Cocoa Nibs	2 tablespoons	Low	Unprocessed chocolate bits, rich in antioxidants and healthy fats
Macadamia Nuts	1 oz	N/A (Low)	High in monounsaturated fats, low in carbs, and a good source of minerals
Sesame Oil	1 tablespoon	N/A (Low)	Adds flavor to dishes and provides healthy fats and antioxidants
Brazil Nuts	1 oz	N/A (Low)	Rich in selenium, healthy fats, and a variety of essential nutrients

Remember to consider portion sizes, monitor blood sugar levels, and consult with healthcare professionals or dietitians for personalized dietary advice.

DAIRY FOODS

Here's a table featuring foods suitable for adults living with diabetes:

Food Type	Portion Size	Low Glycemic Index (GI)	Nutritional Information
Greek Yogurt	1 cup	N/A (Low)	High in protein, probiotics, and calcium
Skim Milk	1 cup	N/A (Low)	Good source of protein, calcium, and vitamin D
Cottage Cheese (Low-Fat)	1 cup	N/A (Low)	Rich in protein, low in carbohydrates, and a source of calcium
Mozzarella Cheese	1 oz	N/A (Low)	Provides protein, calcium, and other essential nutrients
Ricotta Cheese (Part-Skim)	1/2 cup	N/A (Low)	Contains protein, calcium, and various vitamins and minerals
Parmesan Cheese	1 tablespoon	N/A (Low)	High in protein, and calcium, and adds flavor to dishes
Feta Cheese	1 oz	N/A (Low)	Lower in calories than some cheeses provides protein and calcium
Swiss Cheese	1 oz	N/A (Low)	Rich in protein and calcium, lower in sodium

Food Type	Portion Size	Low Glycemic Index (GI)	Nutritional Information
			compared to some cheeses
Cheddar Cheese	1 oz	N/A (Low)	Provides protein, calcium, and essential nutrients
Cream Cheese (Low-Fat)	1 oz	N/A (Low)	Lower in fat compared to regular cream cheese, a source of protein
Butter	1 tablespoon	N/A (Low)	Contains saturated fats, use in moderation
Kefir	1 cup	N/A (Low)	Fermented dairy drink, provides probiotics and some vitamins
Low-Fat Yogurt	1 cup	N/A (Low)	Contains protein, and probiotics, and is lower in fat compared to regular yogurt
String Cheese	1 piece	N/A (Low)	A convenient snack option provides protein and calcium
Cottage Cheese (Full-Fat)	1 cup	N/A (Low)	Rich in protein, and calcium, and a source of healthy fats

Food Type	Portion Size	Low Glycemic Index (GI)	Nutritional Information
Sour Cream (Light)	2 tablespoons	N/A (Low)	Lower in fat than regular sour cream, use in moderation
Blue Cheese	1 oz	N/A (Low)	Intense flavor, adds a tangy taste to salads and dishes
Whole Milk	1 cup	N/A (Low)	Higher in fat, use in moderation, provides protein and calcium
Yogurt Parfait	1 serving	N/A (Low)	Combines yogurt with fruits and granola for a balanced snack
Cottage Cheese with Fruit	1 serving	N/A (Low)	Pairs protein-rich cottage cheese with the natural sweetness of fruits
Cottage Cheese with Nuts	1 serving	N/A (Low)	Combines the protein of cottage cheese with the healthy fats of nuts
Provolone Cheese	1 oz	N/A (Low)	Source of protein and calcium, adds a mild flavor to dishes
Yogurt Smoothie	1 cup	N/A (Low)	Blends yogurt with fruits for a refreshing and nutritious drink

Food Type	Portion Size	Low Glycemic Index (GI)	Nutritional Information
Low-Fat Cream Cheese	1 oz	N/A (Low)	Lower in fat than regular cream cheese, a source of protein
Goat Cheese	1 oz	N/A (Low)	Creamy and tangy, adds a distinct flavor to salads and dishes
Chocolate Milk (Low-Fat)	1 cup	Medium	Provides protein, calcium, and may be enjoyed in moderation
Swiss Cheese and Turkey Roll	1 roll	N/A (Low)	Combines lean protein from turkey with the rich flavor of Swiss cheese
Yogurt with Berries	1 serving	N/A (Low)	Pairs the goodness of yogurt with the natural sweetness of berries
Colby Jack Cheese	1 oz	N/A (Low)	Combines Colby and Monterey Jack cheeses, providing protein and calcium
Chocolate Greek Yogurt	1 cup	Low	Blends the richness of chocolate with the benefits of Greek yogurt

Food Type	Portion Size	Low Glycemic Index (GI)	Nutritional Information
Mexican Cheese Blend	1 oz	N/A (Low)	Combines different cheeses, and adds flavor to Mexican dishes

Remember to choose dairy options that fit your dietary needs, monitor portion sizes, and consult with healthcare professionals or dietitians for personalized dietary advice.

DAIRY ALTERNATIVE FOODS

Here's a table featuring alternative foods suitable for adults living with diabetes:

Food Type	Portion Size	Low Glycemic Index (GI)	Nutritional Information
Almond Milk	1 cup	Low	Low in calories, a source of vitamin E, and may be fortified with calcium
Soy Milk	1 cup	Low	Contains protein, and may be fortified with calcium, vitamin D, and B12

Food Type	Portion Size	Low Glycemic Index (GI)	Nutritional Information
Oat Milk	1 cup	Low	Good source of fiber may be fortified with vitamins and minerals
Coconut Milk (Unsweetened)	1 cup	Low	Rich in healthy fats, may be fortified with calcium
Cashew Milk	1 cup	Low	The creamy texture may be fortified with vitamins and minerals
Rice Milk	1 cup	Medium	Low in fat, may be fortified with calcium and vitamin D
Hemp Milk	1 cup	Low	Contains omega-3 fatty acids, and may be fortified with vitamins and minerals
Flax Milk	1 cup	Low	Rich in omega-3 fatty acids may be fortified with vitamins and minerals
Pea Milk	1 cup	Low	High in protein, may be fortified with calcium, vitamin D, and B12

Food Type	Portion Size	Low Glycemic Index (GI)	Nutritional Information
Greek-Style Almond Yogurt	1 cup	Low	Dairy-free alternative with the consistency of Greek yogurt
Coconut Yogurt	1 cup	Low	Made from coconut milk, rich and creamy consistency
Soy Yogurt	1 cup	Low	Dairy-free alternative made from soy milk contains protein
Oat Yogurt	1 cup	Low	Made from oat milk, may be fortified with vitamins and minerals
Almond-Based Cheese	1 oz	N/A (Low)	Dairy-free cheese alternative made from almonds
Soy-Based Cheese	1 oz	N/A (Low)	Cheese alternative made from soy may be fortified with nutrients
Coconut-Based Cheese	1 oz	N/A (Low)	Cheese alternative made from coconut, with a unique flavor
Cashew-Based Cheese	1 oz	N/A (Low)	Cheese alternative made from cashews, creamy and flavorful

Food Type	Portion Size	Low Glycemic Index (GI)	Nutritional Information
Vegan Cream Cheese	1 oz	N/A (Low)	Dairy-free alternative, often made from soy or nuts
Almond-Based Ice Cream	1/2 cup	Low	Dairy-free dessert option, may be lower in sugar and calories
Coconut-Based Ice Cream	1/2 cup	Low	Creamy and flavorful dessert made from coconut milk
Soy-Based Ice Cream	1/2 cup	Low	Dairy-free dessert option, may be fortified with vitamins and minerals
Oat-Based Ice Cream	1/2 cup	Low	Dessert alternative made from oats, may be lower in fat and calories
Cashew-Based Ice Cream	1/2 cup	Low	Creamy and indulgent dessert made from cashews
Rice-Based Ice Cream	1/2 cup	Medium	Dessert alternative made from rice, may be lower in fat and calories

Food Type	Portion Size	Low Glycemic Index (GI)	Nutritional Information
Almond-Based Yogurt	1 cup	Low	Dairy-free yogurt alternative, may be fortified with nutrients
Coconut-Based Yogurt	1 cup	Low	Yogurt alternative made from coconut milk, creamy and rich
Soy-Based Yogurt	1 cup	Low	Dairy-free yogurt alternative, contains protein and probiotics
Oat-Based Yogurt	1 cup	Low	Yogurt alternative made from oats, may be fortified with nutrients
Cashew-Based Yogurt	1 cup	Low	Creamy yogurt alternative made from cashews
Rice-Based Yogurt	1 cup	Medium	Yogurt alternative made from rice, may be lower in fat and calories
Almond Butter	2 tablespoons	N/A (Low)	Nut butter made from almonds, rich in healthy fats and protein

Food Type	Portion Size	Low Glycemic Index (GI)	Nutritional Information
Cashew Butter	2 tablespoons	N/A (Low)	Creamy nut butter made from cashews, provides healthy fats and protein
Sunflower Seed Butter	2 tablespoons	N/A (Low)	Nut butter made from sunflower seeds, a source of healthy fats
Flaxseed Butter	2 tablespoons	N/A (Low)	Nut butter made from flaxseeds, rich in omega-3 fatty acids
Coconut Butter	2 tablespoons	N/A (Low)	Spread made from coconut flesh, provides healthy fats

When incorporating dairy alternatives into your diet, be sure to check for added sugars and choose options that align with your dietary preferences and health goals. Monitoring portion sizes and consulting with healthcare professionals or dietitians can help ensure a balanced and diabetes-friendly approach.

HERBS AND SPICY FOODS

Here's a table featuring herbs and spices suitable for adults living with diabetes:

Food Type	Portion Size	Glycemic Index	Nutritional Information
Basil	1 tablespoon	Low	Contains vitamins A, K, and antioxidants
Cilantro	1 tablespoon	Low	Rich in antioxidants and may have anti-inflammatory properties
Parsley	1 tablespoon	Low	Contains vitamins A, C, and K, and may support kidney health
Mint	1 tablespoon	Low	Aids digestion, may help alleviate symptoms of irritable bowel syndrome
Rosemary	1 teaspoon	Low	Contains antioxidants and may support brain health
Thyme	1 teaspoon	Low	Rich in antioxidants, may have anti-inflammatory properties
Oregano	1 teaspoon	Low	Contains antioxidants and may have antimicrobial properties
Sage	1 teaspoon	Low	Rich in antioxidants, may support memory function
Dill	1 tablespoon	Low	Contains vitamins A, and C, and minerals like iron and manganese

Food Type	Portion Size	Glycemic Index	Nutritional Information
Chives	1 tablespoon	Low	May have antimicrobial properties and is rich in vitamins
Turmeric	1 teaspoon	Low	Contains curcumin with anti-inflammatory and antioxidant properties
Cinnamon	1 teaspoon	Low	May help regulate blood sugar levels and is rich in antioxidants
Ginger	1 teaspoon	Low	Contains gingerol with anti-inflammatory and antioxidant properties
Garlic	1 clove	Low	May have potential blood sugar-lowering effects and is rich in manganese
Cayenne Pepper	1/4 teaspoon	Low	Contains capsaicin, which may boost metabolism and reduce appetite
Paprika	1 teaspoon	Low	Contains antioxidants and may support cardiovascular health
Coriander	1 teaspoon	Low	May have antimicrobial properties and is rich in vitamins

Food Type	Portion Size	Glycemic Index	Nutritional Information
Fennel Seeds	1 teaspoon	Low	May help regulate blood sugar levels and support digestive health
Cardamom	1 teaspoon	Low	Contains antioxidants and may have anti-inflammatory properties
Nutmeg	1/4 teaspoon	Low	Contains antioxidants and may have anti-inflammatory properties
Cumin	1 teaspoon	Low	May have blood sugar-lowering effects and is rich in iron
Mustard Seeds	1 teaspoon	Low	Contains antioxidants and may have anti-inflammatory properties
Black Pepper	1/4 teaspoon	Low	May improve digestion and enhance nutrient absorption
Cloves	1/4 teaspoon	Low	Contains antioxidants and may have anti-inflammatory properties
Bay Leaves	1 leaf	Low	May have anti-inflammatory and antimicrobial properties

Food Type	Portion Size	Glycemic Index	Nutritional Information
Saffron	1/4 teaspoon	Low	Contains antioxidants and may have mood-enhancing properties
Nutritional Yeast	1 tablespoon	Low	Rich in B vitamins, including B12, and provides a cheesy flavor
Tarragon	1 teaspoon	Low	Contains antioxidants and may have anti-inflammatory properties
Lemongrass	1 stalk	Low	May have anti-inflammatory and antioxidant properties
Chili Powder	1 teaspoon	Low	Contains capsaicin, which may boost metabolism and reduce appetite
Curry Powder	1 teaspoon	Low	Contains various spices with antioxidant and anti-inflammatory properties
Fennel	1 bulb	Low	Rich in fiber, and vitamin C, and may support digestion
Vanilla Extract	1 teaspoon	Low	Adds flavor without added sugars, use in moderation
Szechuan Peppercorns	1 teaspoon	Low	May have anti-inflammatory properties and a unique citrusy flavor

Food Type	Portion Size	Glycemic Index	Nutritional Information
Dulse	1 tablespoon	Low	Seaweed rich in minerals, including iodine, and may support thyroid health
Mace	1/4 teaspoon	Low	Contains antioxidants and may have anti-inflammatory properties
Juniper Berries	1 teaspoon	Low	May have anti-inflammatory and antioxidant properties
Poppy Seeds	1 teaspoon	Low	Rich in manganese, and calcium, and may add a nutty flavor to dishes
Caraway Seeds	1 teaspoon	Low	May aid digestion and provide a source of fiber
Safflower Petals	1 tablespoon	Low	Used for color and may have antioxidant properties
Za'atar	1 teaspoon	Low	Middle Eastern spice blend containing thyme, sesame, and sumac
Allspice	1/4 teaspoon	Low	Contains antioxidants and may have anti-inflammatory properties

Remember to use herbs and spices in moderation, as they can enhance the flavor of dishes without the need for excess salt or added sugars. Consult with healthcare professionals or dietitians for personalized dietary advice.

WATER-BASED FOODS

Certainly! Here's a table featuring water-based foods suitable for adults living with diabetes:

Food Type	Portion Size	Glycemic Index	Nutritional Information
Cucumber	1 cup slices	Low	Low in calories, hydrating, and contains vitamins K and C
Watermelon	1 cup cubes	High	Hydrating, high in vitamins A and C, but consume in moderation due to natural sugars
Celery	1 stalk	Low	Low in calories, hydrating, and a source of fiber
Iceberg Lettuce	1 cup shredded	Low	Hydrating, low in calories, and contains small amounts of vitamins A and K
Radishes	1 cup slices	Low	Low in calories, hydrating, and provides a small amount of fiber
Zucchini	1 cup slices	Low	Low in calories, hydrating, and contains vitamins A and C
Strawberries	1 cup whole	Low	Hydrating, high in vitamin C, and antioxidants

Food Type	Portion Size	Glycemic Index	Nutritional Information
Spinach	1 cup raw	Low	Low in calories, hydrating, and a rich source of vitamins and minerals
Broccoli	1 cup raw	Low	Hydrating, high in fiber, and contains vitamins C and K
Bell Peppers	1 cup slices	Low	Hydrating, rich in vitamins A and C, and provides fiber
Grapefruit	1 medium	Low	Hydrating, rich in vitamins A and C, and contains antioxidants
Cantaloupe	1 cup cubes	Medium	Hydrating, high in vitamins A and C, but consume in moderation due to natural sugars
Cabbage	1 cup shredded	Low	Low in calories, hydrating, and provides fiber
Cauliflower	1 cup raw	Low	Hydrating, low in calories, and contains vitamins C and K
Tomatoes	1 medium	Low	Hydrating, rich in vitamins A and C, and contains antioxidants
Blueberries	1 cup	Low	Hydrating, high in antioxidants, and may have anti-inflammatory properties

Food Type	Portion Size	Glycemic Index	Nutritional Information
Romaine Lettuce	1 cup shredded	Low	Hydrating, low in calories, and provides vitamins A and K
Asparagus	1 cup raw	Low	Hydrating, low in calories, and contains vitamins A and K
Pineapple	1 cup chunks	Medium	Hydrating, contains vitamin C, but consume in moderation due to natural sugars
Oranges	1 medium	Low	Hydrating, rich in vitamin C, and contains fiber
Cabbage	1 cup shredded	Low	Low in calories, hydrating, and provides fiber
Carrots	1 medium	Medium	Hydrating, rich in beta-carotene, and provides fiber
Cucumber	1 cup slices	Low	Low in calories, hydrating, and contains vitamins K and C
Watercress	1 cup raw	Low	Hydrating, low in calories, and a source of vitamins A and C
Kiwi	1 medium	Low	Hydrating, high in vitamin C, and provides fiber
Bell Peppers	1 cup slices	Low	Hydrating, rich in vitamins A and C, and provides fiber
Raspberries	1 cup	Low	Hydrating, high in fiber, and contains antioxidants

Food Type	Portion Size	Glycemic Index	Nutritional Information
Lettuce Wraps	2 large leaves	Low	Use lettuce leaves to wrap fillings for a low-carb, hydrating option
Cranberries	1 cup	Low	Hydrating, high in antioxidants, and may support urinary tract health
Pear	1 medium	Low	Hydrating, provides dietary fiber, and contains vitamins C and K
Coconut Water	1 cup	Low	Natural electrolyte-rich hydration, low in calories

These water-based foods are not only hydrating but also provide essential vitamins and minerals. As with any diet, it's important to monitor portion sizes and consult with healthcare professionals or dietitians for personalized dietary advice.

Chapter 5: Exercise and Physical Activity for Diabetes Management

Diabetes management is a multifaceted journey, and one crucial component of this journey is exercise and physical activity. Engaging in regular physical activity can play a pivotal role in controlling blood sugar levels, improving insulin sensitivity, and enhancing overall well-being. In this chapter, we will delve into the intricacies of the relationship between exercise and diabetes management, exploring the role of exercise in blood sugar control, tailoring exercise routines for diabetes management, and ensuring safe and effective workouts for adults with diabetes.

The Role of Exercise in Blood Sugar Control

Understanding the Mechanisms

Exercise serves as a powerful tool in the arsenal against diabetes by influencing various physiological mechanisms that impact blood sugar control. When we engage in physical activity, our muscles require additional energy, and glucose becomes a primary source. This increased demand for glucose uptake by the muscles contributes to a reduction in blood sugar levels.

Moreover, exercise enhances insulin sensitivity, a crucial aspect for individuals with diabetes. Insulin sensitivity refers to how effectively the body's cells respond to insulin, the hormone responsible for facilitating glucose entry into cells. Regular physical activity helps cells become more responsive to insulin, allowing for improved glucose uptake and utilization.

Additionally, exercise has a sustained impact on blood sugar levels even after the activity concludes. This is due to the continued uptake of glucose by muscles during the post-exercise recovery period. As a result, individuals who incorporate regular exercise into their routine may experience more stable and controlled blood sugar levels over time.

Types of Exercise and Their Effects

Various types of exercises can contribute to blood sugar control in distinct ways. Both aerobic exercises and resistance training offer unique benefits for individuals with diabetes.

Aerobic Exercise: Aerobic or cardiovascular exercises, such as walking, jogging, cycling, and swimming, involve continuous, rhythmic movements that elevate the heart rate and increase breathing. These exercises are particularly effective in improving insulin sensitivity and lowering blood sugar levels.

During aerobic exercise, muscles utilize glucose for energy, reducing the concentration of glucose in the bloodstream. Furthermore, aerobic activities promote cardiovascular health, which is crucial for individuals with diabetes, as they are at a higher risk of cardiovascular complications. Improved cardiovascular health contributes to better overall blood circulation, ensuring that glucose and insulin are efficiently transported throughout the body.

Engaging in regular aerobic exercise can also lead to weight management, another key aspect of diabetes control. Maintaining a healthy weight can enhance insulin sensitivity and reduce the risk of complications associated with diabetes.

Resistance Training: Resistance or strength training involves activities that target specific muscle groups, such as weightlifting or bodyweight exercises. While these activities may not directly lower blood sugar levels during the activity, they play a pivotal role in long-term glucose management.

Muscles developed through resistance training have a heightened capacity to absorb glucose, contributing to improved insulin sensitivity. As these muscles become more metabolically active, they can efficiently utilize glucose for energy, helping to maintain blood sugar within a healthy range.

Moreover, resistance training supports weight management by increasing muscle mass. Lean muscle tissue requires more energy at rest, aiding in the regulation of body weight and contributing to overall metabolic health.

Optimal Duration and Frequency

Determining the optimal duration and frequency of exercise is essential for individuals with diabetes. While the American Diabetes Association recommends at least 150 minutes of moderate-intensity aerobic activity per week, individuals can customize their routines based on their fitness levels, preferences, and health conditions.

Breaking down exercise into manageable sessions throughout the week is often more practical for those new to or returning to physical activity. This could involve 30 minutes of moderate-intensity exercise on most days, which could be further divided into shorter sessions if needed.

For resistance training, incorporating activities targeting major muscle groups at least two days per week is recommended. This could involve using resistance bands, free weights, or engaging in bodyweight exercises. It's crucial to include a variety of exercises to ensure a comprehensive and balanced approach to fitness.

Tailoring Exercise Routines for Diabetes Management

Individualized Approach to Exercise

One of the key principles in effectively managing diabetes through exercise is adopting an individualized approach. Each person's body responds differently to various types and intensities of physical activity, necessitating personalized routines that align with their health status, fitness level, and preferences.

Consultation with Healthcare Professionals: Before initiating any exercise program, individuals with diabetes should consult with their healthcare team. This includes healthcare providers, diabetes educators, and possibly, physical therapists. These professionals can assess the individual's overall health, provide insights into potential exercise-related risks, and offer tailored recommendations.

Healthcare professionals will consider factors such as the individual's age, overall health, existing complications, and medication regimen when devising an exercise plan. This collaborative approach ensures that exercise aligns with the individual's broader healthcare strategy, contributing positively to diabetes management without compromising overall well-being.

Considerations for Blood Sugar Monitoring

Monitoring blood sugar levels before, during, and after exercise is crucial for individuals with diabetes. This practice allows individuals to understand how their bodies respond to different activities and helps in fine-tuning their exercise routines.

Before Exercise: Checking blood sugar levels before starting any exercise provides valuable information about the baseline. It helps individuals make informed decisions about the intensity and duration of the upcoming activity. If blood sugar levels are too high or too low, adjustments to the exercise plan or dietary intake may be necessary.

During Exercise: For longer or more intense activities, periodic checks of blood sugar levels can help prevent extreme highs or lows. Continuous glucose monitoring systems provide real-time data, offering a convenient option for those engaging in prolonged physical activity.

After Exercise: Observing blood sugar levels after exercise helps individuals understand the post-exercise impact on glucose levels. This knowledge aids in adjusting post-workout nutrition, insulin doses, or other aspects of diabetes management.

Adapting to Individual Preferences

Exercise doesn't have to be confined to traditional gym routines. Tailoring exercise to individual preferences increases the likelihood of adherence, fostering a sustainable and enjoyable fitness journey.

Choosing Enjoyable Activities: Whether it's dancing, gardening, hiking, or playing a sport, incorporating activities that bring joy and satisfaction can make exercise a more integral part of daily life. Enjoyable activities are more likely to be sustained in the long run, contributing consistently to diabetes management.

Socializing through Exercise: Engaging in physical activities with friends, and family, or joining group classes not only adds a social element but also provides a support system. Having a workout buddy can make exercise more enjoyable and motivate individuals to stay consistent.

Varied Exercise Modalities: Exploring different types of exercise can prevent monotony and target various muscle groups. Alternating between aerobic exercises, resistance training, and flexibility activities can provide a well-rounded fitness routine.

Safe and Effective Workouts for Adults with Diabetes

Pre-Exercise Precautions

Ensuring the safety and effectiveness of workouts for adults with diabetes involves taking certain precautions, especially when considering the potential impact on blood sugar levels.

Blood Sugar Monitoring and Adjustments: Before starting any exercise, individuals should check their blood sugar levels to ensure they are within a safe range. If levels are too low (hypoglycemia), consuming a small, easily digestible carbohydrate snack can help raise blood sugar. Conversely, if levels are elevated, it may be advisable to delay exercise until they stabilize.

Hydration: Proper hydration is essential before, during, and after exercise. Dehydration can affect blood viscosity and circulation, potentially impacting blood sugar control. Individuals should consume an adequate amount of water based on their activity level and environmental conditions.

Foot Care: Foot care is crucial for individuals with diabetes, as they may be more prone to foot-related complications. Wearing comfortable, well-fitted shoes and checking feet regularly for any signs of injury or infection is essential. Individuals should also avoid exercising barefoot to minimize the risk of cuts or abrasions.

Balancing Medications and Exercise

For individuals taking medications, including insulin or oral hypoglycemic agents, coordinating medication schedules with exercise is critical. Adjustments may be necessary to prevent hypoglycemia during or after physical activity.

Timing of Medications: Discussing the timing of medications with healthcare providers is crucial. For some individuals, taking medications after meals or adjusting doses on exercise days may be necessary to prevent low blood sugar levels.

Carrying Emergency Supplies: Carrying emergency supplies, such as glucose tablets or snacks, is essential during exercise. In the event of hypoglycemia, these supplies can be readily accessible to raise blood sugar levels to a safe range.

Gradual Progression and Warm-Up

Regardless of fitness levels, individuals with diabetes should approach exercise with a focus on gradual progression and proper warm-up routines.

Start Slow and Progress Gradually: Embarking on a new exercise regimen should begin at a comfortable pace, gradually increasing intensity and duration over time. This gradual progression allows the body to adapt to the demands of physical activity, reducing the risk of injuries and complications.

Importance of Warm-Up: Warming up before engaging in more intense exercises is crucial for preventing injuries and ensuring optimal performance. A warm-up increases blood flow to muscles, enhances flexibility, and prepares the cardiovascular system for the upcoming activity.

Incorporating Flexibility and Balance Exercises

While aerobic and resistance training are vital components of a well-rounded exercise routine, flexibility and balance exercises should not be overlooked.

Flexibility Exercises: Stretching exercises enhance flexibility, promoting a full range of motion in joints. Improved flexibility can aid in preventing injuries and contribute to better posture. Yoga and Pilates are examples of activities that incorporate flexibility exercises.

Balance Exercises: Enhancing balance is especially important for individuals with diabetes, as peripheral neuropathy and changes in sensation may increase the risk of falls. Balance exercises, such as standing on one leg or Tai Chi, can improve stability and reduce the risk of injuries.

Post-Exercise Recovery and Monitoring

After completing a workout, individuals should pay attention to post-exercise recovery strategies to ensure a smooth transition and minimize potential complications.

Cool Down: Similar to warm-up routines, cooling down after exercise is crucial. Gradually decreasing the intensity of the activity allows the heart rate to return to baseline and helps prevent dizziness or fainting.

Monitoring for Delayed Hypoglycemia: In some cases, individuals may experience delayed hypoglycemia several hours after exercise. Monitoring blood sugar levels post-exercise and adjusting meals or snacks accordingly can help prevent this phenomenon.

Listening to the Body: Individuals should pay attention to how their bodies respond to exercise. If they experience persistent fatigue, dizziness, or any unusual symptoms, it's essential to consult with healthcare professionals to identify potential issues or adjustments needed in the exercise routine.

Incorporating exercise into the management of diabetes is a dynamic and personalized journey. Recognizing the pivotal role of exercise in blood sugar control, tailoring exercise routines for individual needs, and ensuring safe and effective workouts are essential components of a comprehensive diabetes management plan.

Regular physical activity not only contributes to better blood sugar management but also promotes overall health and well-being. By understanding the mechanisms through which exercise influences blood sugar levels, tailoring routines to individual preferences, and adopting safety measures, individuals with diabetes can embark on a fulfilling and sustainable path toward improved health.

As with any aspect of diabetes management, collaboration with healthcare professionals is paramount. Regular check-ins with healthcare providers, diabetes educators, and other specialists ensure that exercise plans align with overall health goals and contribute positively to the holistic well-being of individuals living with diabetes. By embracing the positive impact of exercise, individuals can take charge of their health, fostering resilience and vitality in the face of diabetes.

Chapter 6: Managing Diabetes in Everyday Life

Living with diabetes requires a multifaceted approach that goes beyond medical interventions. Everyday life involves a myriad of challenges and opportunities, and managing diabetes effectively involves navigating through various aspects of daily living. In this chapter, we will explore essential aspects of managing diabetes in everyday life, including coping with stress and emotional well-being, strategies for dining out and social situations, and tips and precautions for traveling with diabetes.

Coping with Stress and Emotional Well-Being

Understanding the Interplay between Stress and Diabetes

Stress is an inherent part of life, but for individuals living with diabetes, managing stress becomes particularly crucial. The relationship between stress and blood sugar levels is intricate, and understanding this interplay is vital for effective diabetes management.

The Stress Response: When the body perceives a threat or stressor, it initiates the "fight or flight" response. Stress hormones, such as cortisol and adrenaline, are released, leading to increased heart rate, elevated blood pressure, and a surge in energy. While this response is essential for survival, chronic stress can have detrimental effects, particularly for individuals with diabetes.

Impact on Blood Sugar Levels: Stress can impact blood sugar levels in several ways. Firstly, the release of stress hormones can trigger the liver to release glucose into the bloodstream, leading to elevated blood sugar levels. Secondly, stress may influence behaviors and routines, potentially affecting dietary choices, physical activity, and adherence to medication regimens.

Strategies for Stress Management

Effectively managing stress is a crucial aspect of diabetes care. Implementing stress management strategies can positively influence blood sugar control and enhance overall well-being.

Mindfulness and Relaxation Techniques: Practices such as mindfulness meditation, deep breathing exercises, and progressive muscle relaxation can help reduce stress levels. These techniques promote a state of relaxation, counteracting the physiological effects of stress hormones.

Regular Physical Activity: Engaging in regular physical activity not only benefits blood sugar control but also serves as a powerful stress management tool. Exercise releases endorphins, the body's natural stress relievers, and provides an opportunity to unwind and clear the mind.

Social Support: Maintaining a strong support system is essential for managing stress. Connecting with friends, family, or support groups provides an outlet for sharing concerns, receiving encouragement, and fostering a sense of belonging.

Time Management and Prioritization: Effective time management and prioritization can help reduce stress related to daily tasks and responsibilities. Breaking down tasks into manageable steps and focusing on priorities can prevent feelings of overwhelm.

Counseling and Therapy: For individuals facing persistent or overwhelming stress, seeking professional counseling or therapy can be beneficial. Mental health professionals can provide coping strategies, emotional support, and tools for managing stress.

Strategies for Dining Out and Social Situations

Balancing Enjoyment and Diabetes Management

Dining out and social situations are integral parts of life, and individuals with diabetes can navigate these scenarios successfully by adopting practical strategies that balance enjoyment with diabetes management.

Making Informed Food Choices: When dining out, making informed food choices is crucial for maintaining blood sugar control. Opting for lean proteins, vegetables, and whole grains can contribute to a balanced meal. It's helpful to review restaurant menus in advance and consider portion sizes to make more mindful choices.

Carbohydrate Awareness: Being aware of carbohydrate content is particularly important for individuals with diabetes. Carbohydrates significantly impact blood sugar levels, and understanding the carbohydrate content of different foods aids in making appropriate dietary decisions. This includes being mindful of hidden sugars in sauces, dressings, and beverages.

Portion Control: Controlling portion sizes is beneficial for everyone, but it holds particular significance for individuals with diabetes. Managing portion sizes helps regulate calorie intake, which, in turn, affects blood sugar levels. Sharing meals or requesting smaller portions when dining out are effective strategies.

Regular Monitoring and Adjustments: Frequent blood sugar monitoring during and after meals provides valuable insights into how different foods affect blood sugar levels. This real-time feedback allows individuals to make necessary adjustments, such as administering insulin or choosing lower-carbohydrate options.

Pre-planning for Special Occasions: Special occasions and social events often involve unique dietary challenges. Pre-planning for these situations, whether it's bringing a dish to share or having a small, balanced snack beforehand, can help individuals manage their blood sugar levels effectively.

Communication and Advocacy

Effective communication is essential when dining out or navigating social situations. Advocating for one's needs and fostering understanding among friends, family, and restaurant staff can significantly contribute to a positive experience.

Communicating Dietary Needs: Communicating dietary needs is crucial when dining out. Informing restaurant staff about specific dietary requirements, such as avoiding added sugars or requesting modifications, ensures that meals align with diabetes management goals.

Educating Friends and Family: Educating friends and family about diabetes and its dietary implications creates a supportive environment. Loved ones who understand the importance of blood sugar control can actively contribute to creating diabetes-friendly meal options.

Choosing Diabetes-Friendly Restaurants: Selecting restaurants that offer a variety of healthy and diabetes-friendly options makes the dining-out experience more enjoyable. Many restaurants now provide nutritional information, making it easier to make informed choices.

Building a Social Support System: Building a social support system that understands and respects dietary needs is invaluable. Friends and family who are aware of diabetes management considerations can offer encouragement and make social gatherings more comfortable.

Traveling with Diabetes: Tips and Precautions

Ensuring Seamless Diabetes Management While Traveling

Traveling can present unique challenges for individuals with diabetes, but with careful planning and adherence to certain precautions, it is entirely feasible to manage diabetes effectively while exploring new destinations.

Pre-travel Preparations: Before embarking on a journey, individuals with diabetes should undertake thorough pre-travel preparations to ensure a smooth experience. This includes:

- **Medical Check-up:** Schedule a pre-travel medical check-up to ensure that overall health is stable and to address any specific concerns related to travel.

- **Medication and Supplies:** Ensure an adequate supply of diabetes medications, insulin, testing supplies, and any other necessary medical equipment. It's advisable to carry extra supplies in case of unexpected delays.

- **Travel Insurance:** Acquire comprehensive travel insurance that covers medical emergencies, including those related to diabetes management. Familiarize yourself with the policy details and emergency procedures.

- **Physician's Note:** Obtain a note from your healthcare provider detailing your diabetes diagnosis, prescribed medications, and any specific recommendations for managing diabetes during travel.

Managing Medications and Insulin: Effectively managing medications and insulin is crucial while traveling. Here are some considerations:

- **Time Zone Adjustments:** If traveling across time zones, work with your healthcare provider to adjust medication and insulin schedules accordingly. Consistency is key to maintaining blood sugar control.

- **Carrying Medications Onboard:** Keep medications and insulin in your carry-on bag to ensure accessibility. Extreme temperatures in the cargo hold of an aircraft can impact the efficacy of insulin.

- **Storage Precautions:** Ensure proper storage of insulin to maintain its effectiveness. Use a cooler bag with ice packs, especially in warmer climates, and avoid exposing insulin to direct sunlight or extreme temperatures.

Dietary Considerations: Maintaining a diabetes-friendly diet while traveling requires careful planning and flexibility. Consider the following tips:

- **Researching Local Cuisine:** Before arriving at a destination, research the local cuisine and identify diabetes-friendly options. Understanding the typical ingredients used in local dishes can assist in making informed choices.

- **Packing Snacks:** Pack a variety of healthy snacks to have on hand, especially in situations where diabetes-friendly options may be limited. Nuts, seeds, and low-carbohydrate snacks are convenient choices.

- **Hydration:** Staying hydrated is essential for overall health and blood sugar control. Carry a refillable water bottle and aim to drink water regularly, especially in warmer climates or during air travel.

Blood Sugar Monitoring and Emergency Preparedness: Vigilant blood sugar monitoring and emergency preparedness are fundamental aspects of traveling with diabetes. Consider the following precautions:

- **Frequent Monitoring:** Increase the frequency of blood sugar monitoring, especially during periods of travel-related stress or changes in routine. Regular monitoring provides timely insights into blood sugar levels.

- **Emergency Kit:** Pack a diabetes emergency kit containing essential items such as glucose tablets, a glucagon kit (if prescribed), and contact information for emergency healthcare services. Ensure that travel companions are aware of the kit's location.

- **Communication with Travel Companions:** If traveling with others, communicate your diabetes management needs, emergency procedures, and where essential supplies are located. This ensures that companions can assist if necessary.

Adjusting to Local Conditions: Adapting to local conditions, including climate, altitude, and lifestyle, is crucial for effective diabetes management. Here are some considerations:

- **Climate Impact:** Be aware of how climate conditions, such as heat or humidity, may affect blood sugar levels. Stay cool, and hydrated, and take precautions to prevent overheating.

- **Altitude Considerations:** If traveling to high-altitude destinations, be mindful of potential changes in insulin requirements. Consult with your healthcare provider about adjustments to insulin dosages.

- **Local Healthcare Access:** Identify local healthcare facilities and pharmacies at your destination. Have contact information readily available in case of emergencies or unexpected medical needs.

Managing diabetes in everyday life requires a holistic and proactive approach. Coping with stress, navigating dining-out scenarios, and successfully traveling with diabetes are all integral components of this journey. By understanding the interplay between stress and blood sugar levels, adopting effective strategies for dining out, and implementing precautions for travel, individuals with diabetes can lead fulfilling lives while effectively managing their health.

The key lies in a proactive mindset, open communication with healthcare professionals, and a commitment to prioritizing self-care. Through mindful choices, ongoing education, and a resilient approach to challenges, individuals can not only manage diabetes effectively but also thrive in their everyday lives. The journey with diabetes is unique for each person, and by embracing a comprehensive approach, individuals can navigate the complexities with confidence and resilience.

Chapter 7: Preventing and Managing Diabetes Complications

Living with diabetes involves not only managing blood sugar levels but also proactively addressing potential complications that can arise over time. This chapter focuses on key aspects of preventing and managing diabetes complications, with a detailed exploration of foot care to prevent diabetic foot problems, the importance of eye health and regular eye exams, and strategies for managing cardiovascular health and reducing associated risk factors.

Foot Care and Preventing Diabetic Foot Problems
Understanding the Importance of Foot Care

For individuals with diabetes, foot care is not merely a routine aspect of personal hygiene; it is a critical component of diabetes management. Diabetes can affect the nerves and blood vessels in the feet, making them vulnerable to complications. Preventing diabetic foot problems involves a combination of daily foot care practices, regular check-ups, and early intervention to address any issues that may arise.

Daily Foot Care Routine:

1. **Daily Inspection:** Conduct a daily inspection of the feet, checking for any cuts, bruises, redness, or changes in skin color. A handheld mirror can be useful for examining the soles and other hard-to-see areas.

2. **Gentle Cleaning:** Wash the feet daily with lukewarm water and mild soap. Avoid soaking for prolonged periods, as excessive moisture can contribute to skin issues.

3. **Moisturizing:** Apply a moisturizer to keep the skin hydrated, focusing on areas prone to dryness. However, avoid applying moisturizer between the toes to prevent fungal growth.

4. **Trimming Nails Carefully:** Trim toenails straight across and file the edges to prevent ingrown toenails. If unsure or if vision is impaired, seeking professional help for nail care is advisable.

5. **Proper Shoe Selection:** Choose comfortable, well-fitting shoes that provide support and do not cause friction or pressure points. Inspect shoes regularly for any foreign objects, rough seams, or damage.

Regular Check-ups and Professional Care:

1. **Annual Foot Exam:** Schedule an annual foot examination with a healthcare professional, ideally a podiatrist or a healthcare provider experienced in diabetic foot care. This comprehensive examination can identify any potential issues early on.

2. **Neuropathy Assessment:** Regularly assess for neuropathy, a common complication of diabetes affecting nerve function. Symptoms may include tingling, numbness, or pain in the feet. Prompt identification allows for timely intervention.

3. **Blood Flow Evaluation:** Assess blood flow to the feet through tests such as Doppler ultrasound. Poor blood circulation can contribute to delayed wound healing and increase the risk of infections.

4. **Prompt Treatment of Issues:** If any foot issues arise, such as cuts, blisters, or infections, seek prompt medical attention. Early intervention can prevent complications from escalating.

5. **Custom Orthotics:** For individuals with specific foot abnormalities or imbalances, custom orthotic inserts prescribed by a podiatrist can provide additional support and help distribute pressure evenly.

Preventing Diabetic Foot Complications:

1. **Blood Sugar Management:** Maintaining optimal blood sugar levels is foundational to preventing diabetic foot problems. Consistent blood sugar control promotes overall nerve and vascular health.

2. **Regular Exercise:** Engaging in regular physical activity supports blood circulation and helps prevent complications related to poor blood flow to the feet. Exercise also contributes to overall diabetes management.

3. **Avoiding Smoking:** Smoking can further compromise blood circulation, increasing the risk of complications. Quitting smoking is beneficial not only for foot health but also for overall cardiovascular well-being.

4. **Proper Foot Elevation:** Elevate the feet when sitting to encourage blood flow. Avoid prolonged periods of sitting or standing, as both can impact circulation.

5. **Annual Eye Exams:** Regular eye exams can detect any diabetes-related eye complications, allowing for timely intervention to preserve vision.

Eye Health and Regular Eye Exams

Prioritizing Vision Care in Diabetes Management

Diabetes can impact various parts of the body, including the eyes. Diabetic eye complications can lead to serious conditions such as diabetic retinopathy, cataracts, and glaucoma. Regular eye exams are instrumental in detecting these issues early, allowing for intervention to preserve vision and prevent further deterioration.

Importance of Regular Eye Exams:

1. **Early Detection of Diabetic Retinopathy:** Diabetic retinopathy is a common complication that affects the blood vessels in the retina. Regular eye exams enable early

detection of changes in the retina, allowing for timely treatment.

2. **Monitoring for Cataracts:** Diabetes increases the risk of developing cataracts, clouding of the eye's lens. Regular eye exams help monitor for the development of cataracts and guide treatment options if necessary.

3. **Detecting Glaucoma:** Diabetes is associated with an increased risk of glaucoma, a condition characterized by increased pressure in the eye. Regular eye exams include tests for glaucoma, aiding in its early detection and management.

4. **Addressing Diabetic Macular Edema:** Diabetic macular edema is a swelling of the macula, the part of the retina responsible for detailed vision. Regular eye exams can detect signs of macular edema, allowing for appropriate intervention.

Frequency of Eye Exams:

1. **Annual Eye Exams:** Individuals with diabetes should undergo a comprehensive eye exam at least once a year. This frequency allows for the timely detection of changes in eye health.

2. **More Frequent Exams in Certain Cases:** In some cases, healthcare providers may recommend more frequent eye exams, especially if there is existing eye disease or a higher risk of complications.

Self-Care for Eye Health:

1. **Blood Sugar Control:** Maintaining stable blood sugar levels is paramount for preserving eye health. Fluctuations in blood sugar can impact the blood vessels in the eyes, contributing to diabetic retinopathy.

2. **Healthy Diet:** Consuming a nutrient-rich diet with a focus on antioxidants, vitamins, and minerals supports overall eye health. Foods rich in omega-3 fatty acids, such as fish, may offer additional benefits.

3. **Regular Exercise:** Engaging in regular physical activity promotes overall cardiovascular health, which is closely linked to eye health. Exercise supports proper blood circulation to the eyes.

4. **Eye Protection:** Wearing sunglasses that block ultraviolet (UV) rays protects the eyes from sun damage. UV exposure can contribute to the development of cataracts.

5. **Avoiding Smoking:** Smoking is a significant risk factor for various eye conditions, including cataracts and age-related macular degeneration. Quitting smoking is beneficial for overall eye health.

Managing Cardiovascular Health and Reducing Risk Factors

Understanding the Interconnection Between Diabetes and Cardiovascular Health

Cardiovascular health is intricately linked to diabetes, with individuals with diabetes facing a higher risk of cardiovascular complications. Managing cardiovascular health involves addressing risk factors that contribute to heart disease and adopting lifestyle modifications that promote overall well-being.

Risk Factors for Cardiovascular Complications in Diabetes:

1. **High Blood Sugar Levels:** Elevated blood sugar levels can contribute to atherosclerosis, the buildup of plaque in the arteries, increasing the risk of heart disease.

2. **Hypertension (High Blood Pressure):** Diabetes is often associated with hypertension, further amplifying the risk of cardiovascular complications.

3. **Dyslipidemia (Abnormal Cholesterol Levels):** Imbalances in cholesterol levels, including high levels of LDL cholesterol and low levels of HDL cholesterol, contribute to atherosclerosis.

4. **Obesity:** Excess body weight, particularly around the abdominal area, is a significant risk factor for cardiovascular disease in individuals with diabetes.

5. **Smoking:** Smoking is a major risk factor for heart disease, and individuals with diabetes who smoke face an elevated risk of cardiovascular complications.

Lifestyle Modifications for Cardiovascular Health:

1. **Blood Sugar Management:** Maintaining optimal blood sugar levels is fundamental to reducing the risk of cardiovascular complications. Consistent blood sugar control positively impacts overall vascular health.

2. **Blood Pressure Control:** Regular monitoring and management of blood pressure are crucial. Lifestyle modifications, including a heart-healthy diet and exercise, can contribute to blood pressure control.

3. **Cholesterol Management:** Addressing dyslipidemia involves adopting a heart-healthy diet low in saturated and trans fats. Medications may be prescribed when lifestyle modifications alone are insufficient.

4. **Healthy Diet:** Embracing a heart-healthy diet rich in fruits, vegetables, whole grains, lean proteins, and healthy fats supports cardiovascular health. Limiting sodium intake is essential for managing blood pressure.

5. **Regular Physical Activity:** Engaging in regular exercise has numerous cardiovascular benefits. Exercise helps control blood sugar levels, manage weight, and improve overall cardiovascular function.

6. **Smoking Cessation:** Quitting smoking is one of the most impactful measures for reducing the risk of cardiovascular complications. Smoking cessation has immediate and long-term benefits for heart health.

Regular Cardiovascular Check-ups:

1. **Annual Cardiovascular Assessment:** Individuals with diabetes should undergo an annual cardiovascular assessment, which may include tests such as lipid profile, blood pressure measurement, and assessment of overall heart health.

2. **Early Intervention for Risk Factors:** Early identification and intervention for cardiovascular risk factors, such as high blood pressure or abnormal cholesterol levels, can prevent the progression of heart disease.

Medication Adherence:

1. **Prescribed Medications:** Adhering to prescribed medications for diabetes management, blood pressure control, and cholesterol management is crucial. Regular medication reviews with healthcare providers ensure optimal treatment.

2. **Aspirin Therapy:** In some cases, healthcare providers may recommend aspirin therapy to reduce the risk of blood clots and cardiovascular events. However, this should be done under the guidance of a healthcare professional.

Stress Management:

1. **Incorporating Stress-Reducing Activities:** Chronic stress can impact cardiovascular health. Engaging in stress-reducing

activities, such as meditation, yoga, or hobbies, contributes to overall well-being.

2. **Adequate Sleep:** Prioritizing sufficient and quality sleep is essential for cardiovascular health. Lack of sleep can contribute to elevated stress hormones and impact blood pressure.

Preventing and managing diabetes complications involves a comprehensive approach that extends beyond blood sugar control. Foot care, eye health, and cardiovascular health are interconnected aspects that require attention and proactive measures. By incorporating daily foot care routines, prioritizing regular eye exams, and addressing cardiovascular risk factors, individuals with diabetes can significantly reduce the likelihood of complications and maintain a high quality of life.

The key lies in a proactive mindset, regular check-ups with healthcare professionals, and a commitment to a holistic approach to health. By understanding the specific risks associated with diabetes, individuals can take charge of their well-being and navigate their diabetes journey with resilience and confidence. Prevention and early intervention are the cornerstones of effective complication management, empowering individuals to lead fulfilling lives while successfully managing their diabetes.

Chapter 8: Support Systems and Resources for Adults with Diabetes

Living with diabetes involves not only personal management but also tapping into a network of support systems and resources that can enhance the overall quality of care. This chapter delves into the importance of building a diabetes care team comprising doctors, educators, and specialists. It also explores the value of support groups and peer networks, providing a sense of community. Additionally, the chapter emphasizes the significance of accessing diabetes education and community resources, empowering individuals to navigate their diabetes journey with knowledge and resilience.

Building a Diabetes Care Team: Doctors, Educators, and Specialists

The Collaborative Approach to Diabetes Care

The management of diabetes is a multifaceted endeavor that benefits greatly from a collaborative and interdisciplinary approach. Building a comprehensive diabetes care team involves assembling a group of healthcare professionals, educators, and specialists who work together to provide personalized care and support.

Primary Care Physician:

1. **Role in Diabetes Management:** The primary care physician plays a central role in coordinating overall healthcare and managing diabetes. They monitor blood sugar levels, assess overall health, and coordinate with other specialists when necessary.

2. **Regular Check-ups:** Regular visits to the primary care physician are essential for ongoing diabetes management. These visits provide an opportunity to assess blood sugar

control, discuss any concerns, and adjust treatment plans as needed.

Endocrinologist:

1. **Specialized Expertise:** An endocrinologist is a specialist with expertise in hormones, including insulin. For individuals with diabetes, consulting an endocrinologist can provide specialized insights into diabetes management, especially in cases of complex or uncontrolled diabetes.

2. **Treatment Adjustments:** Endocrinologists may make adjustments to medication regimens, and insulin dosages, or recommend advanced therapies to optimize blood sugar control.

Diabetes Educator:

1. **Education and Empowerment:** Diabetes educators are instrumental in providing education and empowering individuals to self-manage their diabetes effectively. They offer insights into lifestyle modifications, medication management, and blood sugar monitoring.

2. **Customized Care Plans:** Diabetes educators work with individuals to create personalized care plans that align with their lifestyle, preferences, and specific needs. This may include dietary guidance, exercise recommendations, and coping strategies.

Registered Dietitian:

1. **Nutritional Guidance:** A registered dietitian specializing in diabetes can offer tailored nutritional guidance. They assist in creating balanced meal plans that support blood sugar control, weight management, and overall well-being.

2. **Carbohydrate Management:** Understanding the impact of carbohydrates on blood sugar levels is crucial, and a dietitian

helps individuals make informed choices while still enjoying a varied and satisfying diet.

Podiatrist:

1. **Foot Health:** Diabetes can impact foot health, and a podiatrist is crucial for preventive care. Regular foot check-ups, nail care, and addressing any issues promptly contribute to preventing diabetic foot complications.

2. **Neuropathy Assessment:** Podiatrists assess for neuropathy, a common complication of diabetes affecting nerve function in the feet. Early identification allows for proactive interventions.

Ophthalmologist:

1. **Eye Health:** Regular eye exams conducted by an ophthalmologist are vital for detecting diabetes-related eye complications such as retinopathy. Early intervention can preserve vision and prevent further deterioration.

2. **Annual Eye Exams:** Individuals with diabetes should undergo annual eye exams to monitor for changes in the retina and other potential eye issues.

Mental Health Professional:

1. **Emotional Well-being:** Managing diabetes involves not only physical but also emotional well-being. Mental health professionals, including psychologists or counselors, can provide support in coping with the psychological aspects of diabetes.

2. **Stress Management:** Addressing stress, anxiety, and depression is crucial for overall diabetes management. Mental health professionals offer strategies to cope with the emotional impact of living with a chronic condition.

Communication and Coordination:

1. **Regular Updates:** Effective communication among members of the diabetes care team is essential. Regular updates and sharing of relevant information ensure that everyone involved is informed about the individual's health status and progress.

2. **Care Coordination Meetings:** Periodic care coordination meetings, where the entire diabetes care team comes together, allow for a comprehensive review of the individual's health, adjustments to the care plan, and addressing any emerging challenges.

3. **Individualized Approach:** The collaborative approach ensures that diabetes management is tailored to the individual's unique needs. A personalized plan takes into account factors such as lifestyle, preferences, and potential challenges.

Support Groups and Peer Networks

The Power of Community in Diabetes Management

Living with diabetes can sometimes be challenging, and the support of peers who share similar experiences can be invaluable. Support groups and peer networks provide a sense of community, understanding, and encouragement that can enhance the emotional and practical aspects of managing diabetes.

Benefits of Support Groups:

1. **Emotional Support:** Sharing experiences with others who understand the challenges of living with diabetes can provide emotional support. Support groups create a space for open dialogue about the highs and lows of managing the condition.

2. **Information Exchange:** Support groups facilitate the exchange of practical tips, strategies, and information related

to diabetes management. Participants can learn from each other's experiences and gain insights into coping mechanisms.

3. **Motivation and Inspiration:** Witnessing the successes and triumphs of others in the group can serve as motivation and inspiration. Seeing individuals successfully navigate diabetes management instills a sense of hope and determination.

4. **Reducing Feelings of Isolation:** Diabetes can sometimes lead to feelings of isolation. Joining a support group helps individuals connect with others facing similar challenges, reducing the sense of isolation and fostering a sense of belonging.

Types of Support Groups:

1. **In-Person Support Groups:** Local community organizations, healthcare providers, or diabetes clinics often organize in-person support groups where individuals can meet face-to-face to share experiences.

2. **Online Support Communities:** Virtual support groups and online communities provide a platform for individuals to connect globally. These platforms offer the flexibility to engage with others at any time, fostering a sense of community.

3. **Specialized Groups:** Some support groups focus on specific aspects of diabetes management, such as those for parents of children with diabetes, individuals managing diabetes and other health conditions, or those interested in specific treatment modalities.

Peer Networks:

1. **Shared Experiences:** Peer networks involve connecting with individuals who are managing diabetes and facing similar

challenges. Sharing experiences and learning from each other creates a sense of camaraderie.

2. **Peer-to-Peer Support:** Peer networks often involve one-on-one support, where individuals can provide encouragement, insights, and practical tips to help each other navigate the complexities of diabetes management.

3. **Local and Global Networks:** Peer networks can exist on both local and global scales. Local networks may involve individuals within a specific community, while global networks connect people from diverse backgrounds.

4. **Online Platforms:** Many peer networks operate through online platforms, allowing individuals to connect regardless of geographical location. Social media groups and dedicated forums provide spaces for ongoing interactions.

Participation and Engagement:

1. **Regular Attendance:** Consistent participation in support groups or peer networks ensures ongoing support and connection with others who understand the journey of managing diabetes.

2. **Active Engagement:** Actively engaging in discussions, sharing personal experiences, and offering support to others create a dynamic and supportive community environment.

3. **Contributing to Discussions:** Individuals can contribute to discussions by sharing tips, and insights, or asking questions. Active participation fosters a collaborative atmosphere where everyone benefits.

4. **Seeking Guidance:** When facing specific challenges or uncertainties, individuals can seek guidance from the collective wisdom of the group. This collaborative problem-solving approach can be empowering.

Empowering Through Knowledge and Outreach

Accessing diabetes education and community resources is fundamental to equipping individuals with the knowledge and tools needed for effective self-management. Educational programs, workshops, and community resources provide valuable insights, practical skills, and a network of support.

Diabetes Education Programs:

1. **Structured Curriculum:** Diabetes education programs often follow a structured curriculum covering various aspects of diabetes management, including nutrition, exercise, medication management, and emotional well-being.

2. **Certified Diabetes Educators (CDEs):** These programs are often facilitated by certified diabetes educators who have specialized training in diabetes care. CDEs guide individuals through the learning process, offering personalized support.

3. **Workshops and Classes:** Diabetes education workshops and classes may cover specific topics such as meal planning, carbohydrate counting, blood sugar monitoring, and stress management. These interactive sessions provide hands-on learning.

Community Resources:

1. **Local Healthcare Providers:** Many local healthcare providers offer diabetes education programs, workshops, and resources. Individuals can inquire about available services through their primary care physician or diabetes care team.

2. **Community Centers and Clinics:** Community centers and clinics often organize health and wellness programs that include diabetes education. These resources may be accessible to individuals within the local community.

3. **Nonprofit Organizations:** Numerous nonprofit organizations focus on diabetes awareness and education. These organizations may provide resources, educational materials, and support for individuals living with diabetes.

4. **Online Platforms:** Online platforms, including reputable websites, forums, and educational portals, offer a wealth of information on diabetes management. These resources may include articles, videos, and interactive tools.

Utilizing Educational Resources:

1. **Attending Workshops and Classes:** Actively participating in diabetes education workshops and classes provides individuals with practical skills and knowledge that can be applied in daily life.

2. **Reading Educational Materials:** Exploring educational materials, such as pamphlets, brochures, and online articles, enhances understanding. Reputable sources, including healthcare organizations and diabetes associations, provide reliable information.

3. **Engaging in Online Learning:** Online learning platforms may offer courses or webinars on diabetes management. These resources allow individuals to learn at their own pace and revisit information as needed.

4. **Connecting with Certified Educators:** Seeking guidance from certified diabetes educators, whether in-person or virtually, ensures that individuals receive accurate and personalized information aligned with their specific needs.

Advocacy and Outreach:

1. **Advocacy for Diabetes Awareness:** Engaging in advocacy efforts for diabetes awareness at the community and societal levels contributes to a broader understanding of the condition and promotes a supportive environment.

2. **Promoting Accessible Resources:** Advocacy can focus on ensuring that educational resources are accessible to all individuals, regardless of socioeconomic status or geographical location. This includes promoting community programs and online resources.

3. **Participation in Supportive Initiatives:** Involvement in community initiatives that promote diabetes awareness, education, and support fosters a sense of belonging and contributes to the well-being of individuals living with diabetes.

4. **Sharing Knowledge:** Individuals who have benefited from diabetes education can become advocates by sharing their knowledge and experiences with others, encouraging them to seek education and support.

Support systems and resources are integral components of effective diabetes management. Building a collaborative diabetes care team ensures that individuals receive holistic and personalized care from healthcare professionals and specialists. Engaging with support groups and peer networks creates a sense of community, fostering emotional well-being and practical insights. Accessing diabetes education and community resources empowers individuals with the knowledge and skills needed to navigate the complexities of diabetes.

By embracing the collective strength of support systems and leveraging educational resources, individuals with diabetes can lead fulfilling lives while effectively managing their health. The journey with diabetes is unique for each person, and by tapping into the wealth of support and knowledge available, individuals can navigate the challenges with resilience, confidence, and a sense of community.

Chapter 9: Thriving with Diabetes: Lifestyle and Self-Care

Living with diabetes is not just about managing the condition; it's about thriving and leading a fulfilling life. This chapter delves into essential aspects of lifestyle and self-care that contribute to thriving with diabetes. Embracing a positive mindset and self-empowerment, understanding the importance of sleep adopting strategies for quality rest, and finding a balance between work, relationships, and diabetes management are key components in the journey towards optimal well-being.

Embracing a Positive Mindset and Self-Empowerment

The Power of Positivity in Diabetes Management

Embracing a positive mindset is a transformative approach that can significantly impact the experience of living with diabetes. A positive outlook not only enhances emotional well-being but also influences physical health and the ability to effectively manage diabetes. Here's a deeper exploration of the importance of a positive mindset and strategies for self-empowerment.

Understanding the Role of Mindset:

1. **Influence on Blood Sugar Levels:** Studies suggest that stress and negative emotions can affect blood sugar levels. Adopting a positive mindset can contribute to better blood sugar control, creating a positive feedback loop for overall health.

2. **Resilience in Facing Challenges:** Living with a chronic condition like diabetes comes with its challenges. A positive mindset enhances resilience, allowing individuals to face challenges with a proactive and solution-oriented approach.

Strategies for Embracing Positivity:

1. **Cultivating Gratitude:** Practicing gratitude involves acknowledging and appreciating the positive aspects of life. Keeping a gratitude journal or simply reflecting on positive moments fosters a sense of well-being.

2. **Mindfulness and Meditation:** Mindfulness techniques, including meditation, can help manage stress and promote a positive outlook. These practices cultivate awareness and allow individuals to stay present, reducing anxiety about the future.

3. **Affirmations:** Positive affirmations involve repeating positive statements to reinforce a positive mindset. Affirmations can focus on strengths, resilience, and the ability to effectively manage diabetes.

4. **Surrounding Yourself with Positivity:** Engaging with positive influences, whether through supportive relationships, uplifting media, or inspiring activities, contributes to maintaining a positive mindset.

5. **Seeking Professional Support:** Mental health professionals, including psychologists or counselors, can provide strategies for managing stress, and anxiety, and maintaining a positive mental outlook.

Self-Empowerment in Diabetes Management:

1. **Setting Realistic Goals:** Establishing achievable and realistic goals in diabetes management builds a sense of accomplishment. Celebrating small victories fosters a positive sense of self-efficacy.

2. **Continuous Learning:** Staying informed about diabetes management, new technologies, and treatment options empowers individuals to actively participate in their care. Knowledge is a powerful tool for self-empowerment.

3. **Effective Communication with Healthcare Team:** Actively engaging with healthcare professionals and communicating openly about concerns, questions, and preferences ensures that individuals actively participate in decisions related to their diabetes care.

4. **Advocating for Personal Needs:** Self-advocacy involves expressing one's needs, preferences, and concerns. Advocating for personalized care and accommodations contributes to a sense of empowerment in diabetes management.

5. **Building a Support System:** Establishing a network of support, including family, friends, and fellow individuals with diabetes, creates a foundation for self-empowerment. Shared experiences and encouragement foster a sense of community.

Overcoming Challenges and Resilience:

1. **Acceptance and Adaptation:** Acceptance of the diagnosis and adapting to the realities of living with diabetes are crucial steps in building resilience. Embracing the journey with openness allows individuals to navigate challenges more effectively.

2. **Learning from Setbacks:** Diabetes management may involve occasional setbacks. Instead of viewing setbacks as failures, reframing them as learning opportunities fosters resilience and a forward-looking perspective.

3. **Celebrating Progress:** Acknowledging and celebrating progress, no matter how small, reinforces a positive mindset. Each step forward is a testament to resilience and the ability to thrive despite challenges.

4. **Fostering a Growth Mindset:** Cultivating a growth mindset involves viewing challenges as opportunities for growth

rather than insurmountable obstacles. This mindset promotes a proactive approach to problem-solving.

5. **Engaging in Hobbies and Passion Projects:** Pursuing hobbies and passion projects provides a sense of fulfillment beyond the realm of diabetes management. Engaging in activities that bring joy contributes to overall well-being.

Sleep and Diabetes: Importance and Strategies for Quality Rest

The Sleep-Diabetes Connection

Quality sleep is a cornerstone of overall health, and its importance is magnified for individuals living with diabetes. The intricate relationship between sleep and diabetes management underscores the need to prioritize restful sleep. This section explores the significance of sleep in diabetes and strategies for achieving quality rest.

Understanding the Sleep-Diabetes Connection:

1. **Impact on Blood Sugar Levels:** Sleep plays a vital role in regulating blood sugar levels. Lack of sleep or poor sleep quality can lead to insulin resistance, impacting blood sugar control.

2. **Hormonal Regulation:** Sleep influences the release of hormones involved in metabolism and appetite regulation. Disrupted sleep patterns can contribute to hormonal imbalances that affect diabetes management.

3. **Link to Insulin Sensitivity:** Adequate sleep promotes insulin sensitivity, allowing the body to use insulin more effectively. This is crucial for individuals with diabetes, as insulin resistance is a common concern.

Strategies for Quality Sleep:

1. **Establishing a Consistent Sleep Schedule:** Going to bed and waking up at the same time every day helps regulate the body's internal clock. Consistency in sleep patterns supports a healthy sleep-wake cycle.

2. **Creating a Relaxing Bedtime Routine:** Engaging in calming activities before bedtime signals to the body that it's time to wind down. This may include activities such as reading, gentle stretching, or practicing relaxation techniques.

3. **Optimizing Sleep Environment:** Creating a comfortable and conducive sleep environment involves factors like room darkness, comfortable bedding, and maintaining a cool temperature. These elements contribute to better sleep quality.

4. **Limiting Screen Time Before Bed:** Exposure to the blue light emitted by screens can interfere with the production of the sleep hormone melatonin. Limiting screen time at least an hour before bedtime supports a night of more restful sleep.

5. **Managing Stress and Anxiety:** Stress and anxiety can disrupt sleep patterns. Adopting stress-reducing practices, such as meditation or deep breathing exercises, helps manage emotional well-being for better sleep.

Diet and Sleep Quality:

1. **Balancing Evening Meals:** Large or heavy meals close to bedtime can disrupt sleep. Balancing evening meals with a combination of carbohydrates, proteins, and healthy fats supports stable blood sugar levels during the night.

2. **Limiting Caffeine and Sugar Intake:** Caffeine and sugar can interfere with sleep. Limiting their intake, especially in the evening, promotes better sleep quality.

3. **Hydrating Mindfully:** Staying hydrated is essential, but excessive fluid intake close to bedtime may lead to disrupted sleep due to trips to the bathroom. Hydrating mindfully earlier in the evening helps avoid this issue.

4. **Considering Evening Snacks:** For individuals with diabetes, a light, balanced snack before bedtime may help stabilize blood sugar levels during the night. Options may include a small portion of protein and complex carbohydrates.

Physical Activity and Sleep:

1. **Incorporating Regular Exercise:** Regular physical activity has numerous health benefits, including improved sleep quality. Engaging in moderate-intensity exercise, such as walking or cycling, contributes to overall well-being.

2. **Timing of Exercise:** While exercise is beneficial, engaging in vigorous activities close to bedtime may have an alerting effect. Planning exercise earlier in the day supports better sleep.

3. **Creating a Relaxing Post-Exercise Routine:** Following exercise with calming activities, such as gentle stretching or a warm bath, signals to the body that it's time to wind down, facilitating the transition to sleep.

Seeking Professional Guidance:

1. **Consulting Healthcare Providers:** If sleep difficulties persist, consulting healthcare providers, including primary care physicians or sleep specialists, is advisable. Identifying and addressing underlying issues is crucial for optimal sleep.

2. **Sleep Studies:** In some cases, healthcare providers may recommend sleep studies to assess sleep patterns and identify potential sleep disorders. These studies provide valuable insights for targeted interventions.

Monitoring Sleep Patterns:

1. **Using Sleep Trackers:** Sleep tracking devices and apps can help individuals monitor their sleep patterns. These tools provide information on factors such as sleep duration, quality, and consistency.

2. **Keeping a Sleep Diary:** Maintaining a sleep diary involves tracking bedtime routines, sleep duration, and any factors that may influence sleep. This diary can be a valuable tool when discussing sleep patterns with healthcare providers.

Balancing Work, Relationships, and Diabetes Management
Integration for Well-Rounded Living

Balancing the demands of work, relationships, and diabetes management is a delicate juggling act that requires intentional effort and effective strategies. Achieving harmony in these aspects of life contributes to overall well-rounded living with diabetes.

Navigating the Workplace:

1. **Open Communication with Employers:** Establishing open communication with employers is essential. Discussing diabetes management needs, such as breaks for blood sugar monitoring or the availability of healthy snacks, fosters a supportive work environment.

2. **Creating a Diabetes-Friendly Workspace:** Individuals with diabetes can optimize their workspace by having easy access to water, healthy snacks, and any necessary diabetes management tools. This ensures a conducive environment for self-care.

3. **Managing Stress at Work:** Workplace stress can impact diabetes management. Implementing stress-management techniques, such as brief breaks for deep breathing or stretching, helps maintain emotional well-being.

4. **Strategies for Long Hours:** For those with demanding work schedules, planning meals and snacks, staying hydrated, and incorporating short breaks for movement support diabetes management during long work hours.

Nurturing Relationships:

1. **Open Communication with Loved Ones:** Openly communicating with loved ones about diabetes management fosters understanding and support. Discussing needs, preferences, and potential challenges ensures a collaborative approach to well-rounded living.

2. **Involving Partners in Meal Planning:** Involving partners or family members in meal planning encourages shared responsibility and promotes a balanced and diabetes-friendly diet for the entire household.

3. **Educating Friends and Family:** Providing friends and family with information about diabetes, its management, and any specific needs helps create an informed and supportive network.

4. **Celebrating Milestones Together:** Celebrating milestones, both related to diabetes management and personal achievements, strengthens relationships and creates a positive environment.

Socializing and Diabetes Management:

1. **Making Informed Choices at Social Events:** Social events often involve food choices that may impact blood sugar levels. Making informed choices, such as opting for healthier options and managing portion sizes, supports diabetes management.

2. **Communicating Dietary Preferences:** Communicating dietary preferences or restrictions to hosts when attending

gatherings ensures that individuals with diabetes have suitable options available.

3. **Carrying Diabetes Supplies:** Being prepared with diabetes supplies, such as medications, blood glucose monitoring tools, and snacks, allows individuals to navigate social situations with confidence.

Quality Time for Self-Care:

1. **Scheduling Dedicated Self-Care Time:** Prioritizing self-care involves scheduling dedicated time for activities such as exercise, relaxation, or pursuing hobbies. This intentional approach ensures that self-care is integrated into daily life.

2. **Setting Boundaries:** Establishing boundaries, whether related to work commitments or personal time, is crucial for maintaining a balance between various aspects of life. Clear boundaries support well-rounded living.

3. **Utilizing Technology for Efficiency:** Technology can streamline various aspects of life. Utilizing apps for meal planning, exercise tracking, and diabetes management can save time and enhance efficiency.

4. **Incorporating Relaxation Techniques:** Managing stress is vital for overall well-being. Incorporating relaxation techniques, such as deep breathing, meditation, or mindfulness, supports emotional health.

Planning for Challenges:

1. **Emergency Preparedness:** Planning for potential challenges, such as unexpected blood sugar fluctuations, ensures that individuals are equipped with the necessary supplies and know how to respond effectively.

2. **Building a Support System:** Having a reliable support system, whether friends, family, or colleagues, assists during

challenging times. Communicating needs and seeking support fosters a collaborative approach to well-rounded living.

Adapting to Life Transitions:

1. **Diabetes Management During Life Changes:** Life transitions, such as moving, changing jobs, or experiencing significant life events, may impact diabetes management. Planning for these transitions and adapting diabetes care accordingly is crucial.

2. **Utilizing Resources for Support:** During major life changes, utilizing available resources, including healthcare providers, support groups, and educational materials, provides additional support for diabetes management.

Thriving with diabetes involves a holistic approach that goes beyond managing blood sugar levels. Embracing a positive mindset and practicing self-empowerment contribute to a resilient outlook on life. Recognizing the importance of quality sleep and implementing strategies for restful nights is integral to overall well-being. Balancing the demands of work, relationships, and diabetes management requires planning and effective strategies for harmonious living.

By integrating these lifestyle and self-care practices, individuals with diabetes can not only manage their condition effectively but also lead fulfilling lives. The journey with diabetes is dynamic and thriving involves adapting to challenges with resilience, fostering positive relationships, and prioritizing self-care. Through a well-rounded approach to lifestyle and self-care, individuals can navigate the complexities of diabetes with confidence, purpose, and a commitment to optimal well-being.

Conclusion: Living a Full and Healthy Life with Diabetes as an Adult

In the grand tapestry of life, the journey with diabetes is but one thread, woven into the rich mosaic of experiences that define who we are. As adults navigating the complexities of this condition, we embark on a path not of limitations but of possibilities—possibilities to lead full, vibrant lives infused with health and well-being.

Our exploration has traversed the realms of understanding diabetes types, causes, and potential complications. We've delved into the intricacies of managing blood sugar levels, from monitoring techniques to medications and insulin therapy. Crafting a diabetes-friendly meal plan became an art, incorporating superfoods and nutrient-rich ingredients to nourish both body and spirit.

The tables we set were not only laden with information but also adorned with an array of non-starchy vegetables, whole fruits, lean proteins, whole grains, healthy fats, dairy, and their alternatives—each a testament to the delectable symphony of choices available to those embracing a diabetes-conscious lifestyle.

Yet, our journey went beyond the plate, venturing into the realms of exercise and physical activity—where the movement became not just a regimen but a celebration of the body's resilience. We strolled through the landscape of everyday life, exploring coping mechanisms for stress, strategies for social situations, and tips for traveling with diabetes.

Preventing and managing complications emerged as a beacon, guiding us to prioritize foot care, eye health, and cardiovascular well-being. Our support systems became pillars of strength, embodying the collaborative spirit of a diabetes care team, the warmth of support groups, and the wealth of knowledge found in education and community resources.

As we unfurled the chapters on lifestyle and self-care, we discovered the art of thriving with diabetes. A positive mindset and self-empowerment became brushstrokes on the canvas of well-being, while the importance of quality sleep and strategies for restful nights illuminated the path to rejuvenation.

Balancing work, relationships, and diabetes management unfolded as a dance—a delicate choreography where each element harmonized to create a well-rounded existence. The finale is a crescendo of a life lived with intention, purpose, and a commitment to holistic health.

So, here we stand at the threshold of possibility, armed not just with knowledge but with the wisdom that living with diabetes is not a constraint but an opportunity. It's an opportunity to savor the vibrant hues of life, to relish the flavors of a well-balanced plate, and to dance to the rhythm of our well-being.

As adults with diabetes, we are not defined by the condition; rather, we define the narrative of our lives. We are the authors, the architects, and the artists of a tale that encompasses resilience, joy, and the relentless pursuit of health. So, let us stride forward, not merely existing but truly living—a symphony of life in which diabetes is but a note, harmonizing with the melody of our journey. May each step be a celebration, and each day an ode to the art of living a full and healthy life with diabetes.

Glossary: Key Terms Related to Diabetes Management

1. **Blood Glucose Monitoring:**

   - *Definition:* The regular checking of blood glucose levels to assess and manage diabetes. It involves using a blood glucose meter to measure the amount of glucose in a small blood sample.

2. **Insulin:**

   - *Definition:* A hormone produced by the pancreas that allows the body to use glucose for energy. In diabetes management, insulin may be administered through injections or an insulin pump to regulate blood sugar levels.

3. **Type 1 Diabetes:**

   - *Definition:* A chronic condition where the pancreas produces little to no insulin. Individuals with Type 1 diabetes rely on insulin injections for survival.

4. **Type 2 Diabetes:**

   - *Definition:* A chronic condition characterized by insulin resistance, where the body's cells do not respond effectively to insulin. It is often managed through lifestyle changes, oral medications, and, in some cases, insulin therapy.

5. **Gestational Diabetes:**

   - *Definition:* Diabetes that occurs during pregnancy. It can increase the risk of complications for both the mother and the baby. Blood sugar levels are usually managed through diet, exercise, and medication if necessary.

6. **HbA1c (Glycated Hemoglobin):**

   - *Definition:* A blood test that measures average blood sugar levels over the past 2-3 months. It is an essential tool for assessing long-term diabetes management.

7. **Carbohydrate Counting:**

   - *Definition:* A method of meal planning that involves tracking the amount of carbohydrates in foods to help manage blood sugar levels. It is commonly used by individuals on intensive insulin therapy.

8. **Hyperglycemia:**

   - *Definition:* High blood sugar levels, often associated with diabetes. It can lead to symptoms such as increased thirst, frequent urination, and fatigue.

9. **Hypoglycemia:**

   - *Definition:* Low blood sugar levels, which can cause symptoms such as shakiness, dizziness, and confusion. It is usually treated with a rapid-acting carbohydrate.

10. **Ketones:**

    - *Definition:* Chemical substances produced when the body breaks down fat for energy. Elevated ketone levels can occur in uncontrolled diabetes and may lead to diabetic ketoacidosis (DKA).

11. **Continuous Glucose Monitoring (CGM):**

- *Definition:* A system that tracks blood sugar levels throughout the day and night. It provides real-time data and alerts for better diabetes management.

12. **Pancreas:**

    - *Definition:* An organ located behind the stomach that produces insulin and other hormones. In diabetes, the pancreas may not produce enough insulin (Type 1 diabetes) or the body may not use it effectively (Type 2 diabetes).

13. **Diabetes Educator:**

    - *Definition:* A healthcare professional with specialized training in diabetes care. Diabetes educators help individuals understand and manage their condition through education and support.

14. **Atherosclerosis:**

    - *Definition:* The buildup of plaque in the arteries, which can lead to cardiovascular complications. Individuals with diabetes are at an increased risk of atherosclerosis.

15. **Peripheral Neuropathy:**

    - *Definition:* Nerve damage that commonly affects the feet and legs. It can cause numbness, tingling, and pain. Diabetes is a common cause of peripheral neuropathy.

16. **Retinopathy:**

    - *Definition:* Damage to the blood vessels in the retina of the eye, leading to vision problems. Diabetic retinopathy is a complication of diabetes that can result in blindness if not managed.

17. **Nephropathy:**

- *Definition:* Kidney damage caused by diabetes. It is a serious complication that can lead to kidney failure if not detected and managed early.

18. **Glucagon:**

- *Definition:* A hormone produced by the pancreas that raises blood sugar levels. It has the opposite effect of insulin and is used in emergencies to treat severe hypoglycemia.

19. **HDL (High-Density Lipoprotein):**

- *Definition:* A type of cholesterol that is considered "good" because it helps remove other forms of cholesterol from the bloodstream. Managing HDL levels is important for cardiovascular health in diabetes.

20. **LDL (Low-Density Lipoprotein):**

- *Definition:* A type of cholesterol that is considered "bad" because it can lead to the buildup of plaque in the arteries. Controlling LDL levels is crucial for cardiovascular health in diabetes.